European School of Oncology

Monographs

Series Editor: U. Veronesi

The European School of Oncology gratefully acknowledges financial support for the Seminar on Familial Cancer Control received from the Swiss Cancer League

Foreword

The European School of Oncology came into existence to respond to a need for information, education and training in the field of the diagnosis and treatment of cancer. There are two main reasons why such an initiative was considered necessary. Firstly, the teaching of oncology requires a rigorously multidisciplinary approach which is difficult for the Universities to put into practice since their system is mainly disciplinary orientated. Secondly, the rate of technological development that impinges on the diagnosis and treatment of cancer has been so rapid that it is not an easy task for medical faculties to adapt their curricula flexibly.

With its residential courses for organ pathologies and the seminars on new techniques (laser, monoclonal antibodies, imaging techniques etc.) or on the principal therapeutic controversies (conservative or mutilating surgery, primary or adjuvant chemotherapy, radiotherapy alone or integrated), it is the ambition of the European School of Oncology to fill a cultural and scientific gap and, thereby, create a bridge between the University and Industry and between these two and daily medical practice.

One of the more recent initiatives of ESO has been the institution of permanent study groups, also called task forces, where a limited number of leading experts are invited to meet once a year with the aim of defining the state of the art and possibly reaching a consensus on future developments in specific fields of oncology.

The ESO Monograph series was designed with the specific purpose of disseminating the results of these study group meetings, and providing concise and updated reviews of the topic discussed.

It was decided to keep the layout relatively simple, in order to restrict the costs and make the monographs available in the shortest possible time, thus overcoming a common problem in medical literature: that of the material being outdated even before publication.

Umberto Veronesi
Chairman Scientific Committee
European School of Oncology

Contents

Treatment

Familial Cancer Control

Participants

Chairmen:

Prof. K. Aoki
Chairman
UICC Epidemiology and
Prevention Programme
President
Aichi Cancer Center
1-1 Kanokoden
Chikusa-Ku
Nagoya 464, Japan

Prof. M. M. Bürger
UICC Treasurer
Chairman
UICC Tumour Biology Programme
Director
Friedrich-Miescher-Institut
P.O. Box 2543
4002 Basel, Switzerland

PD Dr. W. Weber
Medical Oncology
Scientific Secretary
Swiss Cancer League
Monbijoustrasse 61
3001 Bern, Switzerland

Participants:

Dr. D. T. Bishop
Head
ICRF Genetic Epidemiology Laboratory
at the University of Leeds
3K Springfield House
Hyde Terrace
Leeds LS2 9LU, UK

Dr. G. Cristofaro
Director
Hereditary Gastrointestinal
Cancer Prevention Center
Via de Terribile 9
72100 Brindisi, Italy

Dr. P. A. Daly
Medical Oncologist
St. James's Hospital
James's Street P.O. Box 580
Dublin 8, Ireland

Dr. L.-J. D'Orey Manoel
Tr. Abarracamento
Peniche 13–2
1200 Lisboa, Portugal

Prof. W. F. Doe
Division of Clinical Sciences
John Curtin School of Medical Research
P.O. Box 334
Canberra City Act 2601, Australia

Dr. M. Gebhardt
Genetic Epidemiologist
Labor Humangenetik
Dept. Forschung
Kantonsspital
4031 Basel, Switzerland

Dr. R. Gillon
Director
Imperial College Health Service
Visiting Professor in Medical Ethics
St. Mary's Hospital Medical School
14, Princes Gardens
London SW7 1NA, UK

PD Dr. J. Cl. Givel
Service de Chirurgie A
Chuv
1011 Lausanne, Switzerland

Dr. J.-M. Haefliger
Medecin-Chef
Service de Radiotherapie et d'Oncologie
Hôpital
Rue du Chasseral 20
2300 La Chaux-de-Fonds, Switzerland

Mrs. Ch. Harocopos
ICRF Colorectal Cancer Unit
St. Mark's Hospital
City Road
London EC1 V2PS, UK

Dr. F. Joris
Medecin-Chef de l'Institut Central
des Hopitaux Valaisans
Grand-Champsec
1950 Sion, Switzerland

Dr. S. Kubba
Master in Surgery Research Fellow
Clinical Etiology Unit
Heuberg 16
4051 Basel, Switzerland

Prof. H. T. Lynch
Creighton University
School of Medicine
Department of Preventive Medicine and
Public Health
California at 24th Street
Omaha, Nebraska 68178, USA

Prof. P. M. Lynch
Section of Gastrointestinal
Oncology and Digestive Diseases
M. D. Anderson Cancer Center
1515 Holcombe Blvd.
Houston, TX 77030, USA

PD Dr. S. Martinoli
Primario, Reparto di Chirurgia
Ospedale Civico
Via Tesserete 46
6900 Lugano, Switzerland

Dr. R. Meier
Oberarzt Gastroenterologie
Medizinische Klinik
Kantonsspital
4410 Liestal, Switzerland

PD Dr. H. J. Müller
Head
Labor Humangenetik
Dept. Forschung
Kantonsspital
4031 Basel, Switzerland

Prof. J.-J. Mulvihill
Dep. of Human Genetics
University of Pittsburgh
Graduate School of Public Health
130 Desoto Street
Pittsburgh, PA 15261, USA

Dr. V. A. Murday
Consultant Clinical Geneticist
ICRF Genetic Epidemiology Laboratory
at the University of Leeds
3K Springfield House
Hyde Terrace
Leeds LS2 9LU, UK

Dr. S. Narod
Department of Medicine
Division of Medical Genetics
The Montreal General Hospital
1650 Ave Cedar
Montreal, Quebec H3G 1A4, Canada

Dr. T. Nomizu
Director
Department of Surgery
Hoshi General Hospital
2-1-16 Omachi
Koriyama 963, Japan

Prof. G. Noseda
President, Swiss Cancer League
Primario di Medicina
Ospedale della Beata Vergine
6850 Mendrisio, Switzerland

Dr. G. Rennert
Dept. of Community Health
Carmel Hospital
7 Michal Street
Haifa 34362, Israel

Dr. M. Roth
Labor Pneumologie
Zentrum für Lehre und Forschung
Kantonsspital
Postfach
4031 Basel, Switzerland

Dr. R. Scott
Labor Humangenetik
Dept. Forschung
Kantonsspital
4031 Basel, Switzerland

Dr. Chr. Sigg
Dermatology
University of Zürich
Regensbergstrasse 91
8050 Zürich, Switzerland

Dr. R. Sigl
Lawyer
Basel Cancer League
Dufourstrasse 5
4052 Basel, Switzerland

Dr. R. H. Sijmons
Dept. of Medical Genetics
University of Groningen
Faculty of Medicine
Antonius Deusinglaan 4
9713 AW Groningen, The Netherlands

Dr. H. Sobol
Head, Oncology-Genetics Unit
Centre Leon Berard
28, Rue Laennec
69373 Lyon Cedex 08, France

Prof. G. N. Stemmermann
Pathologist, Japan-Hawaii Cancer Study
Kuakini Medical Center
347, North Kuakini Street
Honolulu, Hawaii 96817, USA

Dr. D. J. B. St. John
Director
Department of Gastroenterology
The Royal Melbourne Hospital
Post Office
Melbourne, Victoria 3050, Australia

Mr. H. R. Stoll
Chairman
European Oncology Nursing Society
Isolierstation DIM
Med. Universitätsklinik A
Kantonsspital
4031 Basel, Switzerland

Dr. R. Telhaug
University Hospital
7000 Trondheim, Norway

Dr. Hans F. A. Vasen
Foundation for the Detection of
Hereditary Tumours
University Hospital
Building No. 50
Rijnsburgerweg 10
2333 AA Leiden, The Netherlands

Dr. F. Watanabe
The Second Department of Surgery
Fukushima Medical College
1 Hikarigaoka
Fukushima 960-12, Japan

Introduction

W. Weber

Swiss Cancer League, Bern, Switzerland

This monograph contains the contributions of a two-day seminar on familial cancer which took place in September 1991 in Lugano, Switzerland. It was presented by the Swiss Cancer League to the European School of Oncology on the occasion of its 10th anniversary. The topic chosen is of practical importance for every doctor and has received little attention until now.

All types of cancer show a tendency to aggregate in families. The extent of inherited susceptibility to cancer is currently a matter of special interest. The real challenge of the future appears to be the behavioural and social issues of risk reduction. Understanding the cultural transmission of risk factors in the family may be one of our strongest allies in this field.Cultural transmission can be even stronger than genetic transmission. A dominant trait is expected to affect only half of all offspring, whereas some culturally transmitted characteristics, such as dietary fat intake or smoking habits, may be transmitted to most or even all offspring. Successful intervention affecting such culturally transmitted factors can be much more successful when directed to families rather than individuals.

Introduction to the Seminar

Prof. G. Noseda, President of the Swiss Cancer League

Ospedale della Beata Vergine, Mendrisio, Switzerland

The Seminar on Familial Cancer is the second major event organised by the Swiss Cancer League, in collaboration with the European School of Oncology.

Cancers of most sites show familial site-specific clustering [1,2]. Of all the factors contributing to breast cancer risk, a strong family history of the disease is the most powerful [3]. It is already evident that members of "cancer families" are aware of, and anxious about, their risks [4].

Family studies are a key to the understanding of the genetic and environmental aetiology of chronic disease [5]. Cancer families are human models of susceptibility to neoplasia [6]. There are now blood tests available to help identify which persons do and which do not carry genes predisposing them to familial diseases [7]. Hereditary metabolic variations affecting the metabolism of carcinogens can be identified [8]. High-risk individuals can benefit from screening programmes [7,9,10]. On the basis of the results thereof, intervention trials can be initiated [11].

The purpose of this two-day seminar is to develop strategies for future familial cancer control activities by the Swiss Cancer League in Switzerland and the International Union Against Cancer worldwide. The first day is devoted to the state of the art and to ethics, while during the second day familiar cancer control strategies will be formulated, hopefully to be taken up by the UICC.

REFERENCES

1 Lynch HT, Hirayama T (eds) Genetic Epidemiology of Cancer. CRC Press, Boca Raton 1989
2 Müller HJ, Weber W (eds) Familial Cancer. Karger, Basel 1985
3 Steel M, Thompson A and Clayton J: Genetic aspects of breast cancer. Br Med Bull 1991 (47):504-518
4 Kelly PT: Counselling needs of women with a maternal history of breast cancer. Patient Counselling and Health Education 1980 (2):118-124
5 Dorman JS, Trucco M, La Porte RE, Kuller LH: Family studies: the key to understanding the genetic and environmental etiology of chronic disease? Genet Epidemiol 1988 (5):305-310
6 Li FP: Cancer families: human models of susceptibility to neoplasia - the Richard and Hinda Rosenthal Foundation Award Lecture. Cancer Res 1988 (48):5381-5386
7 Sobol H, Narod SA et al: Screening for multiple endocrine neoplasia type 2a with DNA-polymorphism analysis. N Engl J Med 1989 (321):996-1001
8 Caporaso N, Pickle LW, Bale S, Ayesh R, Hetzel M, Idle J: The distribution of debrisoquine metabolic phenotypes and implications for the suggested association with lung cancer risk. Genet Epidemiol 1989 (6):517-524
9 Vasen HFA, den Hartog Jager FCA, Menko FH, Nagengast FM: Screening for hereditary non-polyposis colorectal cancer: a study of 22 kindreds in the Netherlands. Am J Med 1989 (86):278-281
10 Vasen HFA, Nieuwenhuijzen Krusemann AC et al: Multiple endocrine neoplasia syndrome type 2: the value of screening and central registration. Am J Med 1987 (83):847-852
11 De Cosse JJ, Miller HH, Lesser ML: Effect of wheat fiber and vitamins C and E on rectal polyps in patients with familial adenomatous polyposis. JNCI 1989 (81):1290-1297

Aetiology and Epidemiology

Markovian Models as a Tool in Epidemiology

Martin Gebhardt [1], Mauro Buser [2], Walter Weber [1], Susanna Mosimann [1], Joachim Torhorst [3] and Hansjakob Müller [1]

1 Human Genetics Laboratory, Department of Research, University Hospital, Basel, Switzerland
2 Hoffmann-La Roche, Basel, Switzerland
3 Institute of Pathology, University of Basel, Basel, Switzerland

A common question in epidemiology is whether a particular group exhibits a certain trait more frequently than expected. The group is identified by the exposure to some supposed causal factor. The trait is most often disease, and the expected frequency is that in a control group which is not exposed to the causal factor, but matches the group under study with regard to potentially confounding variables such as age and sex.

In this paper we propose an application of Markovian models to calculate expected frequencies. For example, the approach can be used to answer the simple question whether cancer is observed more frequently in a group of first relatives of a cancer patient than in the general population. However, more complex situations are covered, such as when the frequency of the association between different diseases is of interest and each disease has age- and sex-specific incidence rates, lethalities and recovery probabilities. We explain the principle of Markovian chains in this special context. Then we describe a computer programme which uses the principle to calculate expected frequencies based on general population data. Finally we give an example of a simple application.

Markovian Models

A simple Markovian model is depicted in Figure 1. The boxes stand for the states in which a person of given age and sex can be at some point in time, *t*, with regard to some disease of interest. The arrows show the logically possible transitions that could occur in the interval until the next point in time, $t+1$. Time is measured in some suitable unit. A probability is associated with each transition as shown by the parameters. For example, the parameter i is the probability that a healthy person will get the disease during the next time interval. Under the hypothesis that the person has no increased risk to get the disease due to some environmental exposure or genetic susceptibility, i can be estimated by the age- and sex-specific incidence of the disease in the general population. The other probabilities in this model are recovery rate r, general mortality m, and lethality l, the latter including the disease as a cause of mortality. These probabilities can be taken from general population statistics. There is a chance that the person will remain in the same state

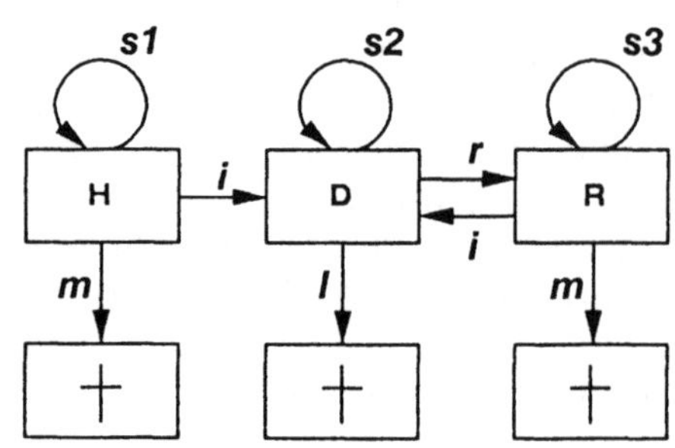

Fig. 1. Simple Markov model with (alive) states "healthy, never diseased" (H), "diseased (D) and "recovered" (R). Each alive state has an associated dead state

during the next time interval. These probabilities (s_1, s_2, s_3) follow from the others because all probabilities associated with the transitions from one state to another (or to itself) must sum up to one. If the person was dead at time t, it is equal to one. There is more than one state labelled "dead" because it may be of interest to separate people who had always been unaffected by a disease from those who were at least once affected.

A model as shown in Figure 1 can be used to describe how the distribution of a cohort of persons changes over time, given that the initial distribution is known. For example, if we start with 1000 healthy persons of the same age and sex, and the probabilities are assumed to be i=0.01, m=0.002 and s_1=0.988, then we expect that after one time step, 988 persons are still healthy, 10 have the disease, and 2 have died. If the probabilities are the same for later time steps, then the same calculations can be repeated as often as necessary, yielding the expected distributions of persons in respective states after subsequent time steps. This is called a stationary Markov chain, because the probabilities are independent of time.

If the probabilities are age-specific, then they will change over time for a cohort of persons. In this instance we have to use a different version of the model for each time step, with changed transition probabilities, but the essential calculations are the same in each step. This is called a non-stationary Markov chain.

Matrix algebra provides a convenient framework to describe Markovian models. At a given time, the distribution of individuals is expressed as a vector **z** with an entry corresponding to each state. The transition probabilities are contained in a square matrix **M** with a row and a column corresponding to each state. For the simple model above we would have (compare also the values from the numerical example):

$$z = [z_H \; z_D \; z_R \; \dot{z}_H \; \dot{z}_D \; \dot{z}_R] = [1000 \; 0 \; 0 \; 0 \; 0 \; 0]$$

$$\mathbf{M} = \begin{pmatrix} s_1 & i & 0 & m & 0 & 0 \\ 0 & s_2 & r & 0 & l & 0 \\ 0 & i & s_3 & 0 & 0 & m \\ 0 & 0 & 0 & 1 & 0 & 0 \\ 0 & 0 & 0 & 0 & 1 & 0 \\ 0 & 0 & 0 & 0 & 0 & 1 \end{pmatrix} = \begin{pmatrix} 0.988 & 0.010 & 0 & 0.002 & 0 & 0 \\ 0 & 0.900 & 0.050 & 0 & 0.050 & 0 \\ 0 & 0.010 & 0.988 & 0 & 0 & 0.002 \\ 0 & 0 & 0 & 1 & 0 & 0 \\ 0 & 0 & 0 & 0 & 1 & 0 \\ 0 & 0 & 0 & 0 & 0 & 1 \end{pmatrix}$$

One can easily verify that the multiplication of the vector with the transition matrix yields the expected state vector for the next time step. The important fact is that with matrix algebra, a Markov chain can be expressed as a simple chain of matrix multiplications, no matter whether we have a simple model such as shown in Figure 1, or a much more complex model where dozens of states could arise, for example, when more than one disease is of interest (e.g., Figs. 2 and 3).

If $\mathbf{z}_t$ is the state vector at time t, and $\mathbf{M}_x$ is the transition matrix for a given age group x, then

$$\mathbf{z}_{t+1} = \mathbf{z}_t\mathbf{M}_x.$$

Following the chain over 2 time steps, and assuming that the transition probabilities change with age, we have

$$\mathbf{z}_{t+2} = \mathbf{z}_{t+1}\mathbf{M}_{x+1} = \mathbf{z}_t\mathbf{M}_x\mathbf{M}_{x+1}.$$

Applying the principle to a cohort born at time t, and following it up to age x, (i.e., up to time t+x), we obtain

$$\mathbf{z}_{t+x} = \mathbf{z}_t\mathbf{M}_1\mathbf{M}_2\mathbf{M}_3...\mathbf{M}_x\,,$$

where $\mathbf{z}_t$ generally has zeroes for all states besides the "healthy" state, because we assume that all persons were initially alive and healthy.

It is easy to see how we can apply the principle to calculate the expected state vector for a sample of persons of mixed ages. First, we have to split the sample into cohorts defined by sensible age classes. Then we calculate the vectors $\mathbf{z}_{t+x}$ for each age class. Finally, we add all resulting vectors together. The procedure amounts to the simulation of the individuals in the sample under the null hypothesis that all transition probabilities are as in the general population. It yields the expected numbers in the different states which can then be compared with the observed numbers by suitable statistical methods.

It should be noticed that with the above procedure it is assumed that the matrix for a given age was constant over the period of calendar time that started with the earliest birth date in the sample. For example, it is assumed that a now 40-year-old and a 60-year-old person experienced the same risk to develop cancer by the age of 30, although the older individual was in the critical age class 20 years earlier than the younger individual. It would be possible in principle to introduce transition matrices that would depend on both age and calendar time without changing the general procedure. The sample would have to be split by age *and* birth date, and different Markov chains would have to be calculated and summed thereafter. The programme described below uses the simpler approach. This limits its application to diseases for which age-specific incidences, lethalities and recovery rates have not substantially changed over the period of time covered by the lives of the persons in the sample.

Computer Programme

A complete Markovian analysis involves 3 main steps: firstly, the model must be specified, including the definition of exclusive states and the assignment of the transition probabilities. Secondly, the expected frequencies have to be calculated for each state. The calculations are based on the data describing the sample (for each individual: sex, age at diagnosis or at death, present state, etc.) and the transition probabilities which are taken from a population based registry. Thirdly, observed and expected frequencies have to be compared with appropriate statistical tests.

The computer programme DISEASES (written by M.B.) performs all these steps automatically according to simple input specifications. Furthermore, it allows to build and maintain a database containing age- and sex-specific data concerning the overall mortality or survival in the general population and data on incidence, recovery, lethality and persistence of codified diseases. The programme has 6 main sections:

1. In the section "Define", the user can specify the size of the time steps between 2 consecutive time points. He can also specify whether the states "affected" or "recovered" should be followed up over more than one transition. This may be desirable if the durations of these 2 states are of interest. For that purpose the programme automatically expands the model by including additional follow-up states as necessary (see Fig. 2). Several diseases can be specified if disease associations or interactions are of interest. The programme expands the model accordingly (Fig. 3).

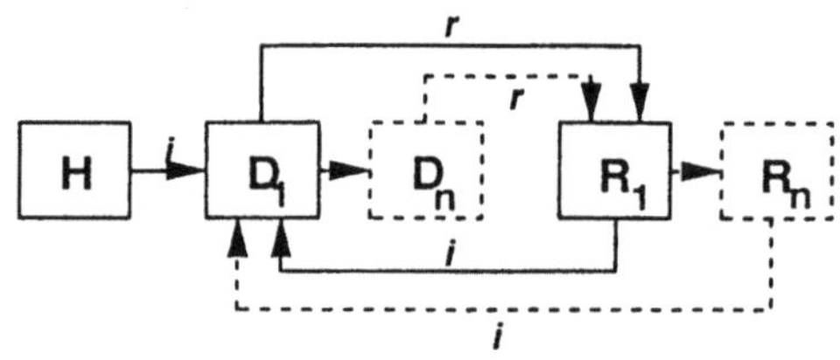

Fig. 2. Expanded Markov model with follow-up of disease and/or recovery. One or more (n) additional states (dashed) are added to the basic model. "Dead" states are not shown for clarity.

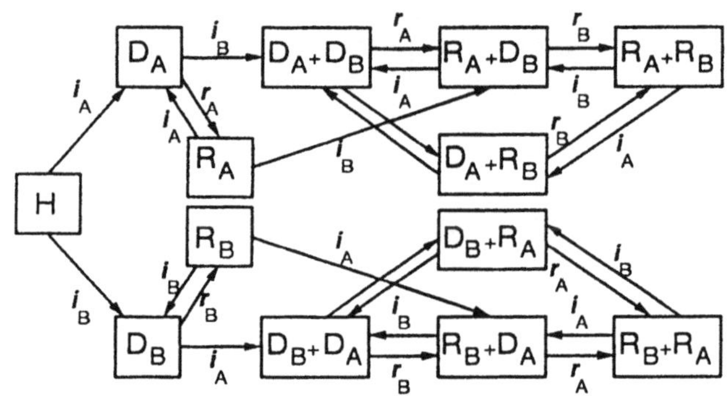

Fig. 3. Markov model for 2 diseases, A and B. It is distinguished whether A follows B or vice versa. "Dead" states and transitions from states to themselves are not shown for clarity.

2. In the section "States", the programme constructs the appropriate Markov model following the instructions given in "Define".

3. In the section "Sample", the user may specify the data describing the sample of individuals, including age or birth date, date of diagnosis, recovery, and so on. It is also possible to specify data windows for ages or calendar time, whether both or a single sex should be analysed, and whether "alive" and "dead" states must be analysed separately.

4. In the section "Loader", the programme reads the data or asks for data missing in the data base. It then amalgamates the probabilities for diseases that have to be grouped together and maps them on the time step size specified.

5. The section "Calcul" performs the matrix multiplications and optionally lists the proba-

bilities for all states in the model by age and sex.

6. The section "Output" prints observed and expected values and their ratio for interesting combinations of states, such as all states involving only one disease, or those involving a specified sequence of states. It also tests the statistical significance of the results. For significant deviations from the expected values, a 95% confidence interval is printed for the ratio of observed and expected frequencies. Three different statistical tests are used according to the magnitude of the expected frequencies. Let E: be the expected frequency, O: the observed frequency and N: the number of individuals in the sample. For $E>5$, the programme compares the statistic

$$\chi^2 = \frac{(|O-E| - 0.5)^2}{E(1-E/N)}$$

to a χ^2 distribution with one degree of freedom. Simulations have shown that this approximation works well in this range. For smaller values of E, the programme compares O with a binomial distribution with parameter E/N, which is a good approximation for $E>2$. For even smaller values of E, the empirical distribution of O is computed by Monte Carlo simulation and used for the statistical test, following a technique described by Wall and Meystre [1].

Example

A detailed family history was obtained from 184 patients (100 men, 84 women) who were diagnosed with non-polyposis colorectal cancer between 1982 and 1988 in Basel. The purpose of the study was to define and quantify tumour associations in the families of the patients. An interview was carried out per-

Table 1. Cancer risk in first relatives of colorectal cancer probands

Cancer	Probands	No. of relatives	No. with cancer	Expected	Relative risk
General	All	1184	162	202.4	0.8 ***
Colorectal	All	1184	39	22.0	1.7 ***
	age<46	90	5	0.9	5.3 **
	46-50	82	2	1.2	1.7
	51-55	157	11	2.0	5.6 **
	56-70	504	12	9.7	1.2
	>70	355	9	8.4	1.1
	with proximal colon cancer	308	15	5.4	2.8 ***
	with distal colon cancer	856	23	16.1	1.4
endometrial	women	(sisters) 296	9	3.1	2.9 **
		(mothers) 181	2	2.9	0.7
stomach	all	1181	21	8.1	2.6 ***
liver	all	1181	6	2.6	2.3 *
lung	all	1181	6	21.3	0.3 ***
prostate	men	581	6	14.0	0.4 *

(Significance: *** $p<0.001$, ** $p<0.01$, * $p<0.05$; otherwise not statistically significant)

sonally by a medical doctor with a standardised questionnaire. All anamnestic data about malignant tumours were verified by medical reports, and by histopathological reports whenever possible. The computer programme DISEASES was used to calculate the probability to be diseased by specified malignancies for each of the 1184 first-degree relatives. Incidence rates were derived rom the population-based Regional Cancer Registry, where 6487 female and 7076 male cases were registered from 1975-1982. Table 1 shows some of the results.

A significantly decreased frequency of malignancies in general was found in the families as compared to the general population. The following malignancies were found in excess: colorectal cancer (especially for young probands and probands with cancer in the proximal colon), endometrial carcinoma (in the sisters only), stomach cancer, and liver cancer. Cancers of the lung and of the prostate gland were significantly under-represented. The apparent deficiency of lung cancers could partly be due to the fact that the incidence of lung cancer has considerably increased over the last decades. Therefore, the relatives spent much of their lives when the incidence in the general population was lower than assumed in the analysis. Since lung cancer is the most common cancer in men, this may also have caused the general deficiency of observed malignancies (indeed, the relative risk for female relatives alone was not significantly different from 1).

REFERENCES

1 Wall M and Meystre M: Testing simple hypotheses by a Monte Carlo-method with sequential decision procedure. Compstat 1974 (74):36-46

Familial Adenomatous Polyposis: Current Status in Switzerland

Rodney J. Scott, Martina Spycher, Walter Weber and Hansjakob Müller

Institute of Human Genetics, Research Department, Kantonsspital Basel, Switzerland

The incidence of Familial Adenomatous Polyposis (FAP) has been shown to be somewhere between 1 in 10,000 and 1 in 20,000 people (taken from the Danish Polyposis Registry). Familial Adenomatous Polyposis is an autosomal dominantly inherited disease characterised by the appearance in the colon of hundreds to thousands of adenomatous polyps at an early age. If left untreated, the disease progresses from the adenomatous stage to adenocarcinoma in virtually 100% of cases. Integrally associated with FAP is a very much severe form of the disease, Gardner's syndrome, which is characterised by desmoid tumors and osteomas. An overview of the known differences between FAP and Gardner's syndrome is shown in Table 1.

Table 1. Clinical features of FAP and Gardner's syndrome

	FAP	Gardner's Syndrome
Osteomas	-	+
Epidermoid cysts	-	+
Polyposis	+	+
Desmoid tumours	+	+
CHRPE*	+	+
Small intestinal carcinomas	-	+
Gastric polyps	-	+
Periampullary carcinomas	+	+
Papillary thyroid carcinoma	-	+
Hepatoblastoma	+	+
Dental abnormalities	-	+

*CHRPE = Congenital Hypertrophy of the Retinal Pigment Epithelium

It has been shown that the disease locus maps to chromosome 5 and more precisely to the region 5q21. Very recently a candidate gene has been described that maps to the 5q21 region and has tentatively been called the APC (or DP 2.5) gene [2-4].

The study of Familial Adenomatous Polyposis in Switzerland began with linkage analysis using the first linked marker to the FAP locus called C11P11. This marker was the same as that described by Bodmer et al. in 1987 [1]. C11P11 was not informative alone for any of the families that we investigated, so further investigations were carried out using probes that were better linked to the FAP locus. A list of current markers that are being studied is shown in Table 2. As can be seen in this Table the relative informativity of these markers alone is not particularly high, however, when used in combination a relative prognosis can be made in such a way that a person at risk can be assigned to a low- or high-risk category.

We have been analysing FAP families from all over Switzerland and have more than 10 verified FAP families that have been or are being investigated. One particularly large family (see Fig. 1) comprising over 300 family members has been of specific interest as it contains both FAP and Gardner's syndrome patients. This family originated in the Puschlav valley and has now spread to nearly all other regions of Switzerland, but concentrates mainly the northwest and the Tessin region.

The index-patient with polyposis coli and cancer of the colon comes from the third generation, branch 2 of this pedigree. It was after this patient's diagnosis that gastroenterological investigations were initiated in

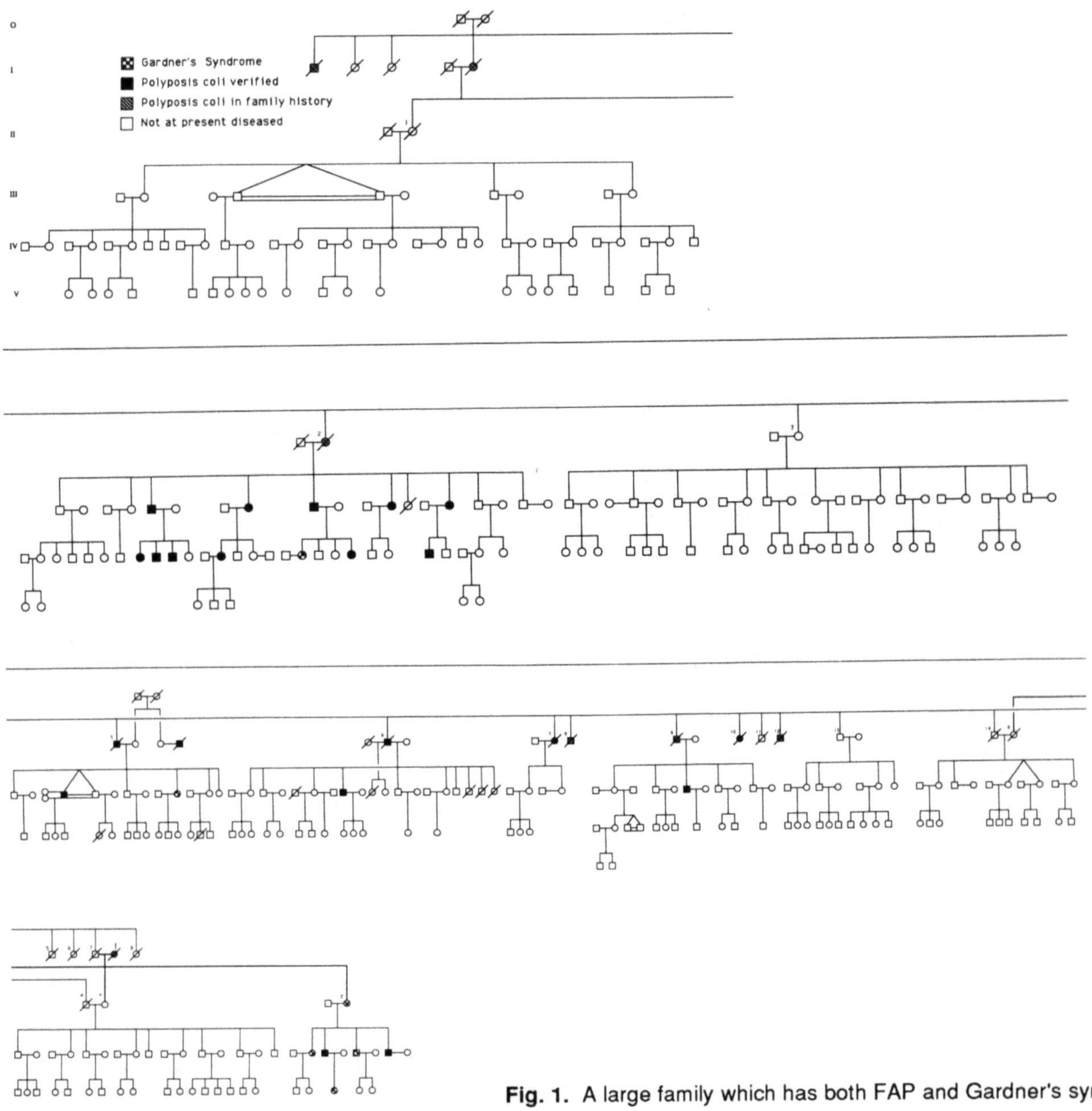

Fig. 1. A large family which has both FAP and Gardner's syndrome

1970 in nearly all siblings. Study of the family revealed a brother suffering from FAP with carcinoma even though the 2 brothers did not know of each other's disease. Further investigations into other branches of the family (III and IV/2 and III and IV/4) led to the identification of other persons affected by FAP or Gardner's syndrome. This family has been and is continuing to be studied by Southern blotting [5] and CA repeat analysis to determine the probability of members being affected by the disease. The presence of congenital hypertrophy of the retinal pigment epithelium (CHRPE) has also been studied in this family and found to be inconsistent as a predictive factor in the assessment of affected individuals.

Since the publication of a likely candidate gene for FAP, we have begun to investigate our families for deletions in the putative FAP gene, looking specifically for mutations within the FAP gene to determine if one or multiple mutations lead to different manifestations of the disease with a view to determining the prognostic outcome of the disease.

Other factors may be involved in the expression of the disease such as the loss of function of the tumour supressor gene p53. This

Table 2. Site-specific polymorphism information content (PIC values) and the recombination fraction of 9 DNA markers that map in the vicinity of FAP

Probe	Polymorphic site	PIC°	Recombination fraction*
p227	Bcl I	0.56	0.05
	Bst XI	0.37	
	Pst I	0.23	
	Mbo I	0.37	
C11P11	Taq I	0.17	0.05
	DEL 1	0.22	
CB26	$(CA)_n$	0.66	
KK5.33	Taq I	0.37	0.07
	Pst I	0.29	
	Bcl I	0.37	
YN5.64	Pst I	0.36	0.06
	Taq I	0.22	
	$(CA)_n$	0.70	
ECB27	Bgl II	0.36	0.05
CB83	Msp I	0.40	0.00
	$(CA)_n$	0.19	
YN5.48	Taq I	0.38	0.01
	Msp I	0.37	
MC5.61	Msp I	0.37	0.04
	Taq I	0.37	

* Recombination fraction estimated by 2-point linkage analysis

° The PIC values indicate the probes' relative usefulness in linkage studies; the higher the number, the more useful the marker. (Taken from the EUROFAP collaborative workshop on FAP, March 1991)

has been shown to occur in adenomas and in adenocarcinomas [6], and it may be a much earlier event in the expression of the disease than originally thought. Additionally, the expression of the disease may be influenced by the transcriptional rate of the FAP gene which could be due to differences in methylation of the promotor sequences of the gene. With these points in mind, we will be in future looking at specific members of our large family to determine what role they play in the expression of FAP and Gardner's syndrome.

REFERENCES

1 Bodmer WF, Bailey C J, Bodmer J et al: Localization of the gene for familial adenomatous polyposis on chromosome 5. Nature 1987 (328):614-616

2 Groden J, Thlivaris A, Samowitz W, Carison M, Gelbert L, Albertson H, Joslyn G, Stevens J, Spirio L, Robertson M, Sargeant L, Krapche K, Wolff E, Burt R, Hughes JP, Warrington J, McPherson J, Wasmuth J, Le Paslier D, Abderrahim H, Cohen D, Leppert M and White R: Identification and characterization of the familial adenomatous polyposis coli gene. Cell 1991 (66):589-600

3 Joslyn, G, Carlson M, Thlivaris A, Albertson H, Gelbert L, Samowitz W, Groden J, Stevens J, Spirio L, Robertson M, Sargeant L, Krapcho K, Wolff E, Burt R, Hughes JP, Warrington J, McPherson J, Wasmuth J, Le Paslier D, Abderrahim H, Cohen D, Leppert M and White R: Identification of deletion mutations and three new genes at the familial polyposis locus. Cell 1991 (66):601-613

4 Kinzler KW, Nilbert MC, Su L-K, Vogelstein B, Bryan T M, Levy DB, Smith KJ, Preisinger AC, Hedge P, McKechnie D, Finnear R, Markham A, Groffen J, Boguski MS, Altschul SF, Horii A, Ando H, Miyoshi Y, Miki Y, Nishisho I and Nakamura Y: Identification of FAP locus genes from chromosome 5q21. Science 1991 (253):661-665

5 Southern EM: Detection of specific sequences among DNA fragments separated by gel electrophoresis. J Mol Biol 1975 (98):503-515

6 Shirasawa S, Urabe U, Yanagawa Y, Toshitani K, Iwama T and Sasazuki T: p53 gene mutations in colorectal tumors from patients with familial polyposis coli. Cancer Res 1991 (51):2874-2878

Down-Regulation of a Cell-Surface Glycoprotein Correlated with Rearrangement of Chromosome 1 in Human Breast Cancer Cells

S. Ashraf Imam [1], Laura A. Mills [1], Sen Pathak [2] and Clive R. Taylor [1]

1 University of Southern California, School of Medicine, Los Angeles, CA 90033, U.S.A.
2 University of Texas, M.D. Anderson Cancer Center, Houston, TX 77030, U.S.A.

The loss of heterozygosity of genes on chromosome 1q, 11p, 13q and 17p in human breast cancer cells has been reported [1-5]. However, reduction to homo- or hemizygosity has not been identified at a molecular level. In the current study, an attempt was made to identify any normal genes that may become inactivated in malignant cells, with associated loss of the gene products.

In order to achieve the above goal, the procedure of tolerisation/immunisation [6] was applied to favour the generation of antibodies to any products present preferentially in normal mammary epithelial cells as compared to their malignant counterparts. Briefly, the tolerance to malignant mammary epithelial cell lines (MCF.7 and MDA.MB.231) was induced in neonatal mice, prior to subsequent immunisation with an extract of normal breast tissue. The tolerised mice, showing absence of serum antibodies against the tolerogen, exhibiting positive reactivity with normal cells, were selected for generating monoclonal antibody. Finally, a monoclonal antibody that exhibited a strong binding with the normal cells, but lacked reactivity against mammary carcinoma cell lines, was selected for further study. The component, detected by the antibody, was termed luminal epithelial antigen (LEA.135).

In order to test the specificity of expression of LEA.135, several human cell lines were used in an indirect immunocytochemical staining method [7]. In addition to employing the widely used lines of malignant mammary epithelial cells, a model system that consists of normal mammary epithelial cell (HMEC), designated 184 [8,9], an immortal cell line (designated 184A1) established from 184 cells by exposure to benzo(a)pyrene [10] and a transformed cell line (designated 184A1N1-T-D10) obtained from 184A1N4, a variant of 184A1, by exposure to oncogenes [11], reflecting various steps of neoplastic transformation, was analysed for the expression of LEA.135. Detailed characteristics of this model system have been described elsewhere [8-11]. Briefly, both the normal (184) and the immortalised (184A1) cells were anchorage dependent for growth, dependent on epidermal growth factor (EGF) for proliferation, and non-tumourigenic in nude mice [8,9]. In contrast, oncogenically transformed cells, derived from the immortalised cells by transformation using retroviral vectors with the oncogene (v-H-ras) and SV40 large T antigen, showed many different growth characteristics [11]. The oncogenically transformed cell line, designated 184A1N4-T-D10, was anchorage independent for growth, independent of EGF as supplement for proliferation, and was tumourigenic in nude mice [8,9]. Unlike the normal or immortalised mammary epithelial cells, the growth of oncogenically transformed 184A1N4-T-D10 was not inhibited by transformation growth factor-beta, TGF-ß [12].

Normal (184) and immortalised (184A1) (Fig. 1) HMEC showed a strong expression of LEA.135 on the surface of their plasma membrane. Application of anti-LEA.135 antibody, preabsorbed with an extract of normal breast cells, failed to react with the target cells (results not shown). In contrast, the oncogenically transformed cell line (184A1N4-T-D10) failed to exhibit a detectable expression of

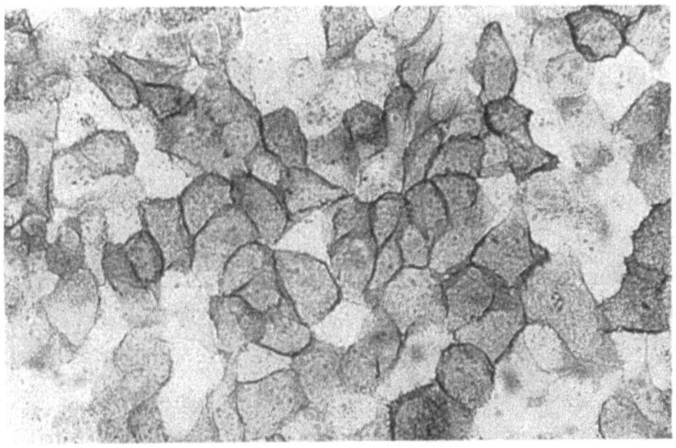

Fig. 1. Preparation and staining of cell lines. The human mammary carcinoma epithelial cell lines (MCF.7 and MDA.MB 231) or normal (184), immortalised (184A1) and oncogenically transformed (184A1N4-T-D10) HMEC were cultured on chamber slides for 3 days, washed with DPBS and fixed with cold-acetone for 30 sec. Biotinylated horse antimouse immunoglobulin was used as the link between the specific antibody and the avidin-biotin-peroxidase complex (ABC). For each experiment, a negative control was performed to ensure the specificity of the reaction; this included use of specific antibody following absorption with extract of the immunogen. Cytopreparation of immortalised HMEC (184A1) was reacted with anti-LEA.135 antibody. The antibody shows strong reactivity predominantly with cell-surface. Original mag. x 200

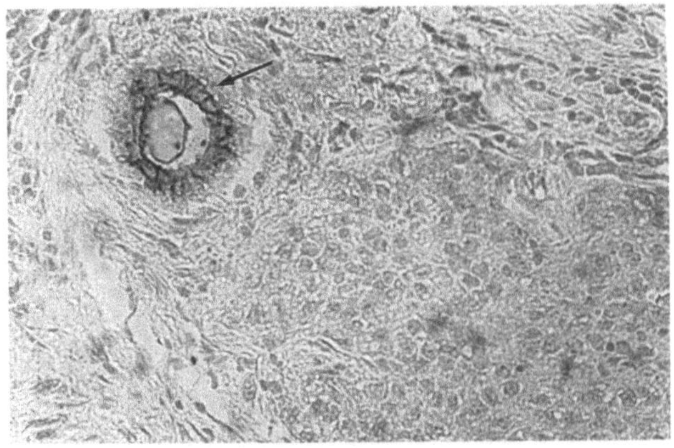

Fig. 2. Preparation and staining of tissue sections. The tissues used were either freshly-frozen in liquid nitrogen or fixed in formalin and embedded in paraffin. The tissues were sectioned at 5 µm, and representative sections were stained with haematoxylin and eosin to confirm the diagnosis prior to immunohistochemical staining. Immunochemical staining of tissue sections was performed as described above (see Legend to Fig. 1). The uninvolved duct at the upper left corner (short arrow) showed strong activity of the cell-surface with the antibody to LEA.135, whereas the surrounding malignant cells (filtrating ductal carcinoma) are non-reactive (original mag. x 320). Reabsorption of anti-LEA.135 antibody with the immunogen led to complete abolition of the staining (results not illustrated). The tissue section was counterstained with Mayer's hematoxylin

LEA.135 (Table 1). In addition, established tumour cell lines that derived from carcinomas of breast (Table 1), cervix, colon, liver, lung, pancreas, kidney, stomach, and thyroid, or melanoma or haematopoietic cell lines (result not shown), also failed to exhibit a detectable amount of LEA.135 expression. The results appear to indicate a correlation between the absence of LEA.135 and the tumourigenicity of *in vitro* HMEC. Furthermore, specificity of expression of LEA.135 on the above breast cell lines was compared with other known epithelial antigens that included human milk-fat-globule membrane antigens, (e.g., epithelial membrane antigen (EMA) [13], human milk-fat-globule membrane glycoprotein (MFGM-gp70) [14,15], MFGM-gp155 [16,17], human milk-fat-globule-1 (HMFG-1) [18], HMFG-2 [19]), epithelial specific pan keratin [20] and receptor for epidermal growth factor (EGF) [21]. In contrast to anti-LEA.135 antibody, antibodies to the above antigens reacted with all the cell lines included in Table 1.

In breast tissues from normal individuals, LEA.135 was expressed predominantly on the apical plasma membrane of luminal epithelial cells lining the ducts (Fig. 2). As in normal breast, benign breast diseases such as fibroadenoma or hyperplasia exhibited the expression of LEA.135. In contrast, invasive mammary carcinoma cells of both infiltrating ductal and infiltrating lobular types failed to exhibit a detectable amount of LEA.135 (Table 2). The results suggest a loss of expression of LEA.135 in invasive primary carcinoma cells of the breast, with the possibility that the gene encoding for LEA.135 may become inactivated during oncogenesis in the breast. A detailed study using a large number of cases is warranted to map more precisely the expression of LEA.135 during the pro-

Table 1. Reactivity of anti-LEA.135 antibody with human mammary epithelial cells by an indirect immunocytological staining method [a]

Cell line	Reactivity with antibody to LEA.135 [b]
184	++
184A1	++
184A1N4-T-D10	-
MCF.7 (oestrogen receptor positive)	-
ZR.75.1 (oestrogen receptor positive)	-
MDA.MB.231 (oestrogen receptor negative)	-
MDA.MB.468 (oestrogen receptor negative)	-

a Samples were scored for intensity on a scale from - to +++: -, absence of staining; +, weak staining; ++, moderate staining; +++, intense staining.

b The cells ($2x10^4$/well) were plated in 0.5 ml of appropriate medium into each well of tissue-culture chambers (Lab. Tek., Nunc, Inc.) and were cultured for 72 hr in a humidified atmosphere containing 5% CO_2. At the end of the incubation period, cells were washed with DPBS and fixed in cold-acetone for 30 sec and stained with anti-LEA.135 antibody using an indirect immunohistochemical method. The antibody preabsorbed with the immunogen served as a control.

gression of breast oncogenesis by incorporating tissue samples from patients with various types of dysplasia and *in situ* carcinoma of breast. In extramammary tissue, a characteristically similar pattern of expression of LEA.135 was also observed in various normal glandular epithelial cells that included cervix, colon, lung, pancreas and stomach. As in breast, the expression of LEA.135 was detectable on the surface of normal cells of the above organs, whereas corresponding malignant epithelial cells in tissue were consistently negative (results not shown). Again, as in cell line, antibodies to other known epithelial antigens failed to discriminate normal from malignant mammary or extramammary epithelial cells in the above tissues.

Table 2. Immunohistological localisation of LEA.135 in formalin-fixed and paraffin-embedded normal or neoplastic breast tissue sections

Histology	No. of specimens studied	No. of specimens stained	Intensity of staining
Normal	10	10	2+ to 3+
Benign	10	10	1+ to 3+
Carcinomas:			
Lobular invasive	10	0	-
Ductal invasive	10	0	-
Medullary invasive	5	0	-
Mucoid invasive	3	0	-
Metastatic to regional lymph node	5	0	-

Histological grading was performed according to the criteria of Bloom and Richardson [22]. Sections were scored for the intensity on a scale from - to 3+: -, absence of staining; 1+, weak staining; 2+, moderate staining; 3+, intense staining

Subsequently, cytogenetics analysis of the cell lines was performed. The widely used cell lines of malignant mammary epithelial cells (MCF.7 and MDA.MB.231, MDA.MB.468 and ZR.75.1) as well as 184A1N4-T-D10 showed a marked rearrangement of its chromosome 1. It is interesting to note that these cell lines were highly tumourigenic and lack the expression of LEA.135. In contrast, immortalised cell line (184A1) which is non-tumourigenic and positive for the expression of LEA.135 exhibited rearrangement in its chromosome 1 (Table 3).

In light of the results obtained, an assay for the expression of LEA.135 may provide a potential means to distinguish normal from malignant and invasive epithelial cells of human breast, and possibly other extramammary organs. Although the significance of expression of LEA.135 and its biological function has yet to be determined, a close correlation was observed between the absence of expression of LEA.135 and the tumourigenicity of oncogenically transformed or established lines of mammary epithelial cells.

Table 3. Determination of tumourigenicity, LEA.135 expression and chromosomes in human mammary epithelial cells

	Cell line tumourigenicity	LEA.135 expression	Chromosome 1 rearrangement
184	-	+	-
184A1	-	+	-
184 B5	-	+	-
184A1N4-T-D10	+	-	+
MCF.7	+	-	+
MDA.MB.231	+	-	+
ZR.75.1	+	-	+

Acknowledgements

We wish to thank Drs. Frank McCormick of Cetus Corporation, Emeryville, CA and Martha R. Stampfer of Lawrence Berkeley Laboratory, University of California, Berkeley, CA, for providing human mammary epithelial cell lines, 184A1N4-T-D10 and 184, 184A1 respectively. We also like to express our thanks to Ms. Sarah and Esther Olivo for skillfully typing the manuscript.

REFERENCES

1 Chen L-C, Dollbaum C and Smith HS: Loss of heterozygosity on chromosome 1q in human breast cancer. Proc Natl Acad Sci USA 1989 (86):7204

2 Genuardi M, Tsihira H, Anderson DE and Saunders GF: Distal deletion of chromosome lp in ductal cancer of the breast. Am J Hum Genet 1989 (45):73

3 Ali IU, Lidereau R, Theillet C and Callahan R: Reduction to homozygosity of genes on chromosome 11 in human breast neoplasia. Science 1987 (238):185

4 Lundberg C, Skooy L, Cavenee WK and Nordenskjöld M: Loss of heterozygosity in human ductal breast tumors indicates a recessive mutation on chromosome 13. Proc Natl Acad Sci USA 1987 (84):2372

5 Mackay J, Elder PA, Steel CM and Forrest APM: Allele loss on short arm of chromosome 17 in breast cancers. Lancet 1988 (ii):1384

6 Imam A, Stathopoulos E and Taylor CR: Generation and characterization of a murine monoclonal antibody to cervical glandular epithelium using mice rendered tolerant to cervical squamous epithelium. Hybridoma 1990 (9):157

7 Imam A, Drushella MM, Taylor CR and Tokes ZA: Generation and immunohistological characterization of human monoclonal antibodies to breast carcinoma cells. Cancer Res 1985 (45):263

8 Hammond SL, Ham RG and Stampfer MR: Serum-free growth of human mammary epithelial cells: rapid clonal growth in defined medium and extended serial passage with pituitary extract. Proc Natl Acad Sci USA 1984 (81):5435

9 Stampfer MR: Isolation and growth of human mammary epithelial cells. J Tissue Culture Methods 1985 (9):107

10 Stampfer MR and Bartley JC: Induction of transformation and continuous cell lines from normal human mammary epithelial cells after exposure to benzo(a)pyrene. Proc Natl Acad Sci USA 1985 (82):2394

11 Clark R, Stampfer MR, Milley R, O'Rouke E, Walen KH, Kriegler M, Kopplin J and McCormick F: Transformation of human mammary epithelial cells by oncogenic retroviruses. Cancer Res 1988 (48):4689

12 Stampfer MR and Bartley JC: Human mammary epithelial cells in culture: differentiation and transformation. In: Dickson R and Lippman M (eds) Breast Cancer: Cellular and Molecular Biology. Martinus Nijhoff, Norwell, MA 1988

13 Heyderman E, Steele K and Ormerod MG: A new antigen on the epithelial membrane: its immunoperoxidase localization in normal and neoplastic tissue. J Clin Pathol 1979 (32):35

14 Imam A, Laurence DJR and Neville AM: Isolation and characterization of a major glycoprotein from milk-fat-globule membranes of human breast milk. Biochem J 1981 (193):47

15 Imam A, Taylor CR and Tokes ZA: Immunohistochemical study of the expression of human milk-fat-globule membrane, glycoprotein 70. Cancer Res 1984 (44):2016

16 Imam A, Laurence DJR and Neville AM: Isolation and characterization of two individual glycoproteins from human milk-fat-globule membranes. Biochem J 1982 (209):37

17 Imam A, Drushella MM, Taylor CR and Tokes ZA: Preferential expression of a Mr 155,000 milk-fat-globule membrane glycoprotein on luminal epithelium of lobules in human breast. Cancer Res 1986 (46):6374

18 Arklie J, Taylor-Papadimitriou J, Bodmer W, Egan M and Millis R: Differentiation antigens expressed by epithelial cells in the lactating breast are also detectable in breast cancers. Int J Cancer 1981 (28):23

19 Burchell J, Wang D and Taylor-Papadimitriou J: Detection of the tumor associated antigens recognized by the monoclonal antibodies HMFG-1 and 2 in serum from patients with breast cancer. Int J Cancer 1984 (34):763

20 Schlegel R, Banks-Schlegal S, McLeod JA and Pinkus GS: Immunoperoxidase localization of keratin in human neoplasms. Am J Pathol 1980 (101):41

21 Sainsbury JRC, Sherbet GV, Farndon JR and Harris AL: Epidermal-growth-factor receptors and oestrogen receptors in human breast cancer. Lancet 1985 (1):364

22 Bloom HJG and Richardson W: Histological grading and prognosis in breast cancer. Br J Cancer 1975 (11):359

Gastric Cancer in Hawaii Japanese: A Family Study

Grant N. Stemmermann

Japan-Hawaii Cancer Study, Kuakini Medical Center, Honolulu, Hawaii, U.S.A.

Gastric cancer incidence and mortality rates have declined throughout western Europe over the past 50 years [1]. The rates in Japan remain high, but appear to be falling. Stomach cancer rates among Hawaii Japanese are now midway between those of the U.S. whites and Japan [2]. These events appear to result from the influence of causal and protective environmental events on stomach cancer risk [3-5]. Familial gastric cancer [6-9] could be heritable or due to a shared environment. The following observations hint at a genetic influence: 1) Pernicious anaemia, a gastric cancer precursor, follows a pattern of autosomal Mendelian transmission [10]; 2) Blood type A predominates in patients with diffuse gastric cancer [11], contrasting with the intestinal type predominating in high-risk populations [12]; 3) Antral gastritis in Colombia has shown Mendelian transmission of a recessive autosomal gene [13]; 4) Some strains of rats are resistant to experimental gastric carcinogens [14]. We have studied a cohort of Hawaii Japanese men since 1965-68. This report assesses the weight of environment and genetics upon stomach cancer in this population.

Methods

The subjects were Japanese men, born between 1900 and 1919, and living in Hawaii. They were identified in 1965 with the use of Selective Service draft registration files [15]. Out of 11,136 men, 8006 (71.9%) were interviewed and examined from 1965-68, 180 (1.6%) died before they could be examined and 2950 (26.5%) did not participate in the programme. The examination included a medical and social history, family history, anthropomorphic measurements, a 24-hour dietary recall, and measurement of serum lipids [15]. From 1971-75, the cohort was re-examined as were 2553 additional men [16]. The latter were brothers not included in the initial examination. Index cases were subjects who developed stomach cancer subsequent to examination. If more than one brother developed stomach cancer during the follow-up period, the brother with the earliest accession was the designated index case. Deaths in primary relatives with no ascertainable cause were arbitrarily classified as tumour free. These were usually parents or older siblings who died in Japan. The study has identified parents, siblings, and children of index cases as follows: 1) Successive questionnaires in the 1965-68 and 1971-74 examinations; 2) this was supplemented by a state population file maintained by the Department of Genetics, University of Hawaii [17]. A total of 6558 families have been identified. The Honolulu hospitals are surveyed on a daily basis for cancer deaths and diagnoses. The Hawaii Tumor Registry identifies cancers missed by this surveillance. Cancers diagnosed before the establishment of the Hawaii Tumour Registry in 1960 were identified from death certificates for the period 1919 to 1942, and from the state population file (see above). The index cases in this analysis were divided into two groups: 1) Families in which the index case was the only gastric cancer - sporadic cancers; 2) Families with stomach cancer affecting at least one primary relative in addition to the index case.

Table 1. Gastric cancer in Hawaii Japanese families

	Gastric cancer	Other GI* cancer	All other cancer	Total
Index Cases	232 (100%)	22 (9.4%)**	23 (9.9%)**	232 (100%)
Parents	58 (12.5%)	14 (3%)	22 (4.7%)	464 (100%)
Fathers	34 (14.7%)	7 (3%)	13 (3.6%)	232 (100%)
Mothers	24 (10.3%)	7 (3%)	9 (3.9%)	232 (100%)
Siblings	36 (3.3%)	34 (3.1%)	74 (6.8%)	1082 (100%)
Brothers	20 (3.2%)	20 (3.2%)	45 (7.3%)	618 (100%)
Sisters	16 (3.4%)	14 (3.0%)	29 (6.3%)	464 (100%)
Children	1 (0.2%)	3 (0.5%)	13 (2.1%)	622 (100%)
Sons	1 (0.3%)	2 (0.6%)	6 (1.8%)	335 (100%)
Daughters	0	1 (0.3%)	7 (2.4%)	287 (100%)

* Small intestine, colon, rectum, liver, gallbladder, bile ducts, pancreas

** Includes all other primary cases found among men identified as index cases of stomach cancer

Results

The frequency of gastric and other cancers in these families is shown in Table 1. Gastric cancer exceeded all other gastrointestinal tumours by about four times among parents of index cases, and approximately equalled the sum of all other gastroenterological (GI) tumours in siblings. The mean age, at diagnosis, of men with sporadic gastric cancer and those from families with multiple gastric cancers was virtually identical: 69.8 and 69.6. The frequency of different histologic types of gastric cancer was similar for both groups. Sporadic cases were intestinal in type in 93/145 cases (64.1%), diffuse in 34 (23.5%) and mixed I/D in 18 (12.4%). The others were intestinal in 50 of 75 cases (66.7%), diffuse in 16 (21.3%) and mixed in 9 (12.0%). A larger proportion of relatives in families with more than 2 stomach cancers had cancers in other GI sites than were found in relatives of men with sporadic cancer (Table 2), but the difference was not significant ($p = 0.2$). Index cases from families with more than 2 stomach cancers were more likely to have been current smokers than men with sporadic cancer (50.7% vs 36.1%, $p = 0.05$). There were 45 separate primary cancers in sites other than the stomach in 39 of the 232 index men with stomach cancer (16.8%). The colon was the most common site of multicentric cancers, and men in the familial group accounted for 8 of 12 of these tumours. Of 20 male siblings with gastric cancer, 4 also had cancers at other sites: colon, lung, urinary bladder and prostate.

There were 16 families with 3 or more gastric cancers (0.2% of 6558 families). Some were noteworthy. The index case in Family No. 701 had colon cancer 10 years prior to the diagnosis of primary cancers of the stomach and duodenum; and autopsy discovered stage 4 prostate cancer. Three siblings had gastric cancer. His father had colon cancer, and one brother had multicentric large bowel cancers. Family No. 7755 had 6 members with gastric cancer, one having colon cancer as well. Two members of this family - a sister and brother - had multiple primary cancers. Family No. 1305 had a father and 2 brothers with gastric cancer, a brother with adrenocortical cancer, and another with lymphosarcoma and metastatic adenocarcinoma from unknown primary site. Another family had 3 gastric cancers and a male sibling with nasopharyngeal cancer (NPC). Breast cancer was found in 8 sisters and 3 daughters of the 232 index men, or in 1.5% of 751 female siblings and children. Only 2 breast cancers were found in the 16 families with 3 or more stomach cancers.

Table 2. Frequency of cancer at non-gastric GI sites and non-GI cancers among relatives of men with sporadic gastric cancer and those from families with multiple gastric cancers

Cases - No.	No. other GI cancers (%)	No. other cancers (%)
Sporadic stomach cancer		
Parents - 314	7 (2.2%)	19 (6%)
Siblings - 672	20 (3.0%)	47 (7%)
Children - 437	3 (0.2%)	11 (2.5%)
TOTAL - 1423	30 (2.1%)	77 (5.4%)
Multiple stomach cancer		
Parents - 150	7 (4.7%)	6 (4%)
Siblings - 410	16 (3.9%)	32 (7.8%)
Children - 185	0	2 (1%)
TOTAL - 745	23 (3.1%)	40 (5.4%)

Discussion

The definition "cancer family" used by the International Collaborative Group on Hereditary Non Polypous Colon Cancer (HNPCC), requires 3 relatives with colorectal cancer, and at least one diagnosed before 50 years of age. Multiple primary cancers also characterise heritable cancer [18]. The similarity of age, histologic cancer type and cancer stage among index men in kindreds with sporadic or multiple gastric cancer may stem from the permissive definition of multiple cancer in our study. The parents and siblings in families with 2 or more gastric cancers, however, did have more frequent cancers of the non-gastric GI tract. This finding, together with more frequent smoking by the index men in these families suggests interaction between the environment and genetics.

Some of these families appeared to be at equal risk of both gastric and large bowel cancer, replicating observations that gastric cancer occurs with increased frequency in relatives of colon cancer patients [18,19]. Colon cancer in this cohort is associated with sedentary lifestyle, weight gain since age 25, and alcohol intake as a percent of total calories, and low calcium intake [20,21]. Stomach cancer is also related to smoking [22], salt intake [5], processed meats [3]. The increase in colon cancer among Hawaii Japanese men coincides with a decrease in gastric cancer. Second generation Japanese gastric cancer rates approach those of U.S. whites, with persisting high rates in first generation migrants [23]. The increased frequency of colon cancer affects both first and second generation men. An excess of both tumours in one family could be explained by a genetic defect common to the all GI cells, but triggered by different environmental events occurring at different times.

Oestrogen and progesterone receptors have been found in gastric cancer from male and female patients [24,25]. It is not likely that oestrogens promoted gastric cancer in our families since they showed no excess of breast cancer, either in the group as a whole, or in the families with 3 or more gastric cancers.

In summary, gastric cancer is familial (i.e., 3 or more per family) in a small number (0.2%) of Hawaii Japanese kindreds. Affected families show an excess of other GI cancers, particularly of the colon. This concurrence could be explained by the interaction of a genetic defect with environmental exposures occurring at different points in time.

REFERENCES

1 Muir CS, Malhotra A: Changing patterns of cancer incidence in five continents. In: Kurihara M (ed) Changing Cancer Patterns and Topics in Cancer Epidemiology. Gann Monograph in Cancer Research, No. 33, Plenum Press, New York 1987

2 Tominaga S: Cancer incidence in Japanese in Japan, Hawaii and Western United States. Fourth Symposium on Epidemiology and Cancer Registries in Pacific Basin. NCI Monograph 69 (Henderson BE, chairman). NIH Publication No 85-2768, Bethesda, MD 1985

3 Nomura A, Hiroshi Y, Ishidate T, Kamiyama S, Masuda H, Stemmermann G, Heilbrun L, Hankin J: Intestinal metaplasia in association with diet. JNCI 1982 (68):401-405

4 Kodama M, Kodama T, Suzuki H, Kondo K: Effect of rice and salty diet on the structure of the mouse stomach. Nutr Cancer 1984 (6):135-147

5 Stemmermann G, Haenszel W, Lacko F: Epidemiologic pathology of gastric ulcer and carcinoma among Japanese in Hawaii. JNCI 1977 (58):13-20

6 Graham S, Lilienfeld AM: Genetic studies of gastric cancer in humans: an appraisal. Cancer 1958 (11):945-959

7 Woolf CM, Isaacson EA: An analysis of 5 "stomach cancer families" in the state of Utah. Cancer 1960 (14):1005-1016

8 Jackson CE, Brownlee RW, Schuman BM, Micheloni F, Ghironzi G: Observations on gastric cancer in San Marino. Cancer 1980 (45):599-602

9 Lehtola J: Family study of gastric carcinoma. Scand J Gastroent 1978 (13, (Suppl. 50):1-54

10 Kekki M, Siurala M, Varis K, Sipponen P, Sistone P, Nevanlinna HR: Classification of principles and genetics of chronic gastritis. Scand J Gastroent 1987 (22,Suppl. 141):1-28

11 Correa P, Sasano N, Stemmermann G, Haenszel W: Pathology of gastric carcinoma in Japanese populations: comparisons between Miyagi Prefecture, Japan, and Hawaii. JNCI 1973 (51):1449-1459

12 Hanai H, Fujimoto I, Taniguchi H: Trends of stomach cancer incidence and histologic types in Osaka. In: Magnus H (ed) Trends in Cancer Incidence. Hemisphere Publishing Corp, Washington 1982 pp 143-154

13 Bonney GE, Elston RC, Correa P, Haenszel W, Zavala D, Zarama G, Collazos T, Cuello C: Genetic etiology of gastric carcinoma: chronic atrophic gastritis. Genet Epidemiol 1986 (3):213-224

14 Ohgaki H, Kawachi T, Matsukura N, Morino K, Miyamoto M, Sugimura T: Genetic control of susceptibility of rats to gastric carcinoma. Cancer Res 1983 (43):3663-3667

15 Kagan A, Harris BR, Winkelstein W, Johnson KG, Kato H, Syme SE, Rhoads G, Gay M, Nichaman MZ, Hamilton HB, Tillotson JL: Epidemiologic studies of coronary heart disease and stroke in Japanese men living in Japan, Hawaii and California. J Chron Dis 1974 (27):345-364

16 Heilbrun LK, Kagan A, Nomura A, Wasnich RD: The origins of epidemiologic studies of heart disease, cancer and osteoporosis among Hawaii Japanese. Haw Med J 1985 (44):294-296

17 Mi MP, Earle M, Kagawa J: Phenotypic resemblance in birth weight between first cousins. Ann Human Gen 1986 (50):49-62

18 Lynch HT, Kimberling W, Albino WA, Lynch JF, Biscone K, Schuelke GS, Sanberg AA, Lipkin M, Deschner EE, Mikol YB, Elston RC, Barley-Wilson JE, Danes BS: Hereditary non polyposis colorectal cancer (Lynch Syndrome I & II), Part I - Clinical description of resource. Cancer 1985 (56):934-938

19 Sondergaard JO, Bulow S, Lynge E: Cancer incidence among parents of patients with colorectal cancer. Int J Cancer 1991 (47):202-206

20 Stemmermann GN: Geographic epidemiology of colorectal cancer. In: HK Seitz, UA Simanowki, NA Wright (eds) Colorectal Cancer: From Pathogenesis to Prevention. Springer-Verlag, Berlin 1989 pp 3-23

21 Stemmermann GN: Prospective study of alcohol intake and large bowel cancer. Dig Dis Sci 1990 (55):1414-1420

22 Nomura A, Grove JS, Stemmermann GN, Severson RK: A prospective study of stomach cancer and its relation to diet, cigarettes and alcohol consumption. Cancer Res 1990 (50):627-631

23 Kolonel LN, Nomura AMY, Hirohata T, Hankin JH, Hinds HW: Association of diet and place of birth with stomach cancer incidence in Hawaii Japanese and Caucasians. Am J Clin Nutr 1981 (34):2478-2485

24 Kojima O, Takahashi T, Kawakami S, Uehara Y, Matsui M: Localization of estrogen receptors in gastric cancer using immunohistochemical staining of monoclonal antibody. Cancer 1991 (67):2401-2406

25 Tokunaga A, Nishi K, Matsukura N, Tanaka N, Onda M, Shirota A, Asano G, Hayashi K: Estrogen and progesterone receptors in gastric cancer. Cancer 1986 (57):1376-1379

Increased Number of Multiple Melanomas in Sporadic and Familial Variants of Dysplastic Naevus Syndrome

Christian Sigg

Institute of Dermatohistopathology, Zürich, Switzerland

In the past decade, a new cancer-associated genodermatosis has been defined, the so-called Dysplastic Naevus Syndrome (DNS) or familial atypical multiple mole melanoma syndrome (FAMMM) [1,2]. This dominant trait with extensive heterogeneity and variable expression shows clinical and histological features characterised by its name: FAMMM is characterised by the association of melanomas affecting several members of a family and the presence of dysplastic naevi. Apart from the inherited variant of DNS there also exists a sporadic form: the frequency of sporadic dysplastic naevi appears to be 2-7% in white adults in the USA. In the Swiss population, DNS was found in 2.5% of men aged 20 and in 7% of patients attending dermatological clinics because of pigmented moles [3,4]. Remarkably, in a study including 939 schoolchildren, clinically defined dysplastic naevi were observed in 2.7%; although histological examination did not confirm all conditions for dysplastic naevus, the melanonaevocytic status of these children (fair skin complexion, increased total number of acquired naevi and increased number of irregular naevi) is strongly suggestive of an early stage of DNS in childhood [5].

Because of the lack of adequate genetic investigations, the number of sporadic cases of DNS has probably been overestimated. Sporadic cases may far exceed familial cases due to the inappropriate use of the term "sporadic".

Cancer-associated genodermatoses are characterised by an early age at cancer onset while having an increased tolerance for cancer when compared to the natural history of sporadic forms. In hereditary cancer syndromes, the tumours are usually not of a single type but of multiple types in different organs. Patients with familial DNS and their relatives not only have an increased incidence of cutaneous malignant melanomas, but also of breast cancer, cancer of the respiratory, gastrointestinal, lymphatic and probably urogenital systems [6-8]. Since it is known that atypical germ cells of the testis occur more frequently in patients with disturbed fertility, it seems remarkable that in our own study on 612 infertile men DNS was found in as many as 6.7% [9].

Besides the sporadic forms, familial forms are present in 1-11% of all malignant melanomas. The familial type of malignant melanoma, however, is heterogeneous and not clearly defined. Three groups of familial malignant melanomas may be distinguished: malignant melanoma without additional skin disorders, melanoma associated with disturbances of the pigmentary system (including albinism, congenital naevi, and DNS) and malignant melanoma in other forms of genodermatosis. The most frequent variant of familial malignant melanoma is DNS.

If DNS really represents an increased tumour risk of the melanonaevocytic system, it is to be expected that patients with this cutaneous phenotype - especially in familial variants - develop not only single but also multiple melanomas.

In our study of 280 melanoma patients (Fig. 1), all data concerning familial and personal history, histology, and therapy were verified. All patients underwent total body skin examination to check the presence of DNS. In 257/280 patients (91.8%), solitary melanomas were found, while in 23/280

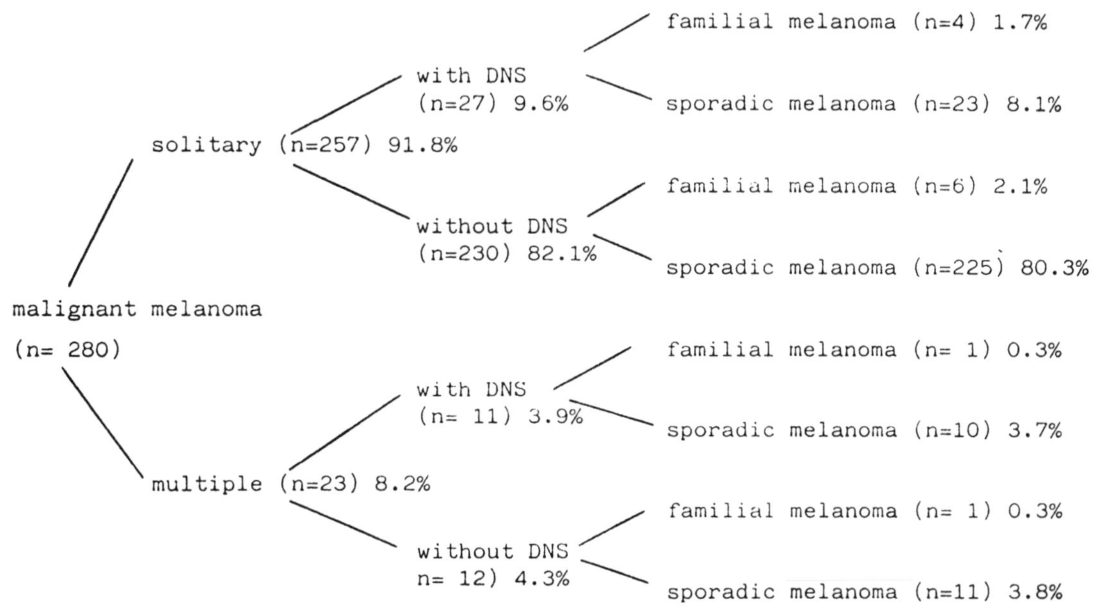

Fig. 1. Relative frequency of solitary and multiple melanoma in patients with and without DNS

patients (8.2%), multiple melanomas occurring simultaneously or consecutively were found. Surprisingly, among the 12/280 patients (4.2%) with familial variants of melanoma, there was no increased frequency of multiple melanomas. In patients with DNS (either sporadic or familial) the frequency of multiple melanoma was higher: in patients with solitary melanomas, DNS was found in 27/257 (10.5%), while in patients with multiple melanomas, DNS was diagnosed in 11/23 (47.8%) ($p = 0.0005$). In both groups (solitary and multiple melanomas) the mean age of patients with DNS was around 10 years lower. The frequency of additional primary malignancies in patients with cutaneous melanomas was 8.6%, and did not vary among patients with solitary or multiple melanomas with or without DNS [10].

In the family history of all melanoma patients, malignant tumours were found in 55.3%. The most frequent were stomach cancer (16.6%), breast cancer (14.7%), skin cancer (12.4%), cancer of the respiratory system (7.7%) and of the lymphatic system (6.5%). Malignant tumours were more frequent in families with sporadic or familial DNS (72%) than in families of patients without DNS (51.4%).

Multiple melanomas of the skin occur more frequently in patients with DNS, regardless of whether they represent sporadic or familial variants. Since melanomas in patients with DNS seem to occur earlier in life, the presence of DNS probably triggers the malignant transformation.

REFERENCES

1 Clark W, Reimer R, Greene R, Ainsworth A, Mastrangelo M: Origin of familial malignant melanoma cases from hereditable melanocytic lesions. Arch Dermatol 1978 (114):732-738

2 Lynch H, Frichot B, Lynch J: Familial atypical multiple mole-melanoma syndrome. J Med Genet 1978 (15):352-356

3 Sigg C, Pelloni F: Frequency of acquired melanonevocytic nevi and their relationship to skin complexion in 939 schoolchildren. Dermatologica 1989 (179) 123-128

4 Sigg C, Pelloni F: Hautstatus und Häufigkeit von Dermatosen bei 603 Rekruten der schweizer Armee. Schweiz Z Milit Med 1990 (67):23-28

5 Sigg C, Pelloni F, Schnyder UW: Increased number of acquired melanonevocytic nevi and atypical appearance of nevi in children. Possible indications of the early stage of dysplastic nevus syndrome in childhood (in press)

6 Lynch HT, Fusaro RM, Pester J, Oosterhuis JA, Went LN, Rumke P, Neering H, Lynch JF: Tumor spectrum in the FAMMM syndrome. Br J Cancer 1981 (44):533-540

7 Lynch HT, Frichot BC, Lynch P, Lynch JF, Guirgis HA: Family studies of malignant melanoma and associated cancer. Surg Gynecol Obstet 1975 (141):517-522

8 Sigg C, Pelloni F: Dysplastic nevi and germ cell tumors of the testis - a possible further tumor in the spectrum of associated malignancies in dysplastic nevus syndrome. Dermatologica 1988 (176):109-110

9 Sigg C: Increased number of DNS and other disturbances of melanonevocytic system in infertile men (in preparation)

10 Sigg C, Pelloni F, Schnyder UW: Gehäufte Mehrfachmelanome bei sporadischem und familiärem dysplastischen Nävuszellnävus-Syndrom. Hautarzt 1989 (40):548-552

Family History in Clinical Trials: Experience of the IBCSG and the SAKK

Monica Castiglione-Gertsch

SIAK/IBCSG Coordinating Centre, Bern, Switzerland

Improved survival, early age at presentation and a high frequency of multiple primary cancers have been reported in patients with a hereditary or familial form of cancer.

Patients included in clinical trials follow selection criteria rules, which generally exclude those with a previous history of cancer and those with multiple cancers, for example women with bilateral breast cancer. The frequency of familiality among patients treated in the context of clinical trials is therefore likely to be lower than in the cancer population of interest. Clinical trials are therefore an inadequate context in the study of incidence of familial cancer.

The follow-up data which is usually generated in a clinical trial and the careful monitoring of the patients is a context in the study of outcome in subsets of patients with or without family history. In addition, patients included in clinical trials belong to a well defined population in terms of prognostic factors, which should allow for discriminaion of the impact of family history upon outcome.

The Swiss Group for Clinical Cancer Research (SAKK) and the International Breast Cancer Study Group (IBCSG) have conducted only a few trials where the study of familiality was one of the purposes. One of the possible explanations for this apparently scarce interest in familiality is surely the fact that the collection of data on family history may be very time consuming in the context of a clinical trial, where the clinician is already faced with the burden of extra work required to complete the documentation of the course of the disease, the treatment, and its toxicity.

Material and Methods

The SAKK is currently conducting a clinical trial evaluating a short adjuvant perioperative chemotherapy regimen given either intravenously or intraportally in radically operated colorectal cancer patients. For this study there is a log of patients diagnosed with the same disease but not included in the trial for various reasons.

Data on family history are collected from all patients, and as of September 1991 data on family history were available for 393 patients of the therapeutic study and for 890 in the log of ineligible patients.

From 1978 to 1985 the IBCSG conducted 5 clinical trials studying adjuvant therapy in operable breast cancer, and data on family history are available for 1086 women included in these studies.

Results

SAKK-Study on Colorectal Cancer

1) More than 10% of patients under the age of 50 have a positive family history for colorectal cancer (we have analysed only first-degree relatives); for patients above 50 this percentage is about 7%.

This indicates the first difficulty when trying to study family history in a clinical trial. Are these percentages real or do they only reflect bad interviewing techniques to the disadvantage of older patients? Or do older patients have more difficulty in recalling the medical histories of their relatives?

A higher percentage of familial cancer in younger people would correspond to most reports in the literature.
2) Males less frequently report a family history for colorectal cancer than females. Women more often describe cancer in other localisations in their family than men. It is questionable whether this is a real finding or a result obtained by chance. Women generally are assumed to be better informed than men about their family and familial diseases.
3) Patients with blood group B and with negative Rhesus factor more frequently report a positive family history than patients with other blood groups or those with positive Rhesus factor.

Family history and patient characteristics (SAKK 40/87)

	Total Nr of pts	None	Colorectal cancer only	Colorectal and other cancers	Other cancers only
Age					
< 50 years	49	33	5 (10.2%)	0	11 (22.4%)
≥ 50 years	344	246	22 (6.4%)	3	73 (21.2%)
Sex					
Female	163	116	6 (3.7%)	1 (0.6%)	40 (24.6%)
Male	230	163	21 (9.1%)	2 (0.9%)	44 (19.1%)
Blood group					
0	164	122	13 (7.9%)	0	29 (17.7%)
A	189	128	10 (5.3%)	0	49 (25.9%)
B	26	17	3 (11.5%)	1 (3.8%)	5 (19.2%)
AB	14	12	1 (8.3%)	0	1 (8.3%)
Rhesus factor					
+	329	235	19 (5.8%)	3 (0.9%)	72 (21.9%
-	64	44	8 (12.5%)	0	12 (18.7%)

IBCSG Studies I-V in early breast cancer

LUDWIG STUDIES I - IV

STUDY DESIGN

STUDY I:	S		R	
	U		A	CMF x 12
	R	PRE- AND PERI-	N	
	G	MENOPAUSAL	D	
	E	1-3 AXILL. NODES	O	CMFp x 12
	R	POSITIVE	M	
	Y			
STUDY II:	S		R	
	U		A	CMFp x 12
	R	PRE- AND PERI-	N	
	G	MENOPAUSAL	D	
	E	4 AND MORE	O	OOPHORECTOMY
	R	AXILL. NODES POS.	M	+ CMFp x 12
	Y			

STUDY III:	S		R	
	U		A	SURGERY ALONE
	R	POSTMENOPAUSAL	N	
	G	NODE POSITIVE	D	CMFp+TAM x12
	E	< 66 YEARS	O	
	R		M	p + TAM x 12
	Y			

STUDY IV:	S		R	
	U		A	SURGERY ALONE
	R	POSTMENOPAUSAL	N	
	G	NODE POSITIVE	D	
	E	66-80 YEARS	O	p + TAM x 12
	R		M	
	Y			

LUDWIG STUDY V

	N-	N+
perioper. CT	-	-
perioper. CT	-	6 x CMF oral
no perioper. CT	-	6 x CMF oral TAM for post

In these studies the characteristics of all the patients included were similar to those reporting a positive family history for first-degree relatives (96 patients), to those with a positive family history for second degree relatives (63 patients) and to those with no family history of breast cancer (927 patients). Outcome was similar for the 3 groups of patients. Disease-free survival curves for studies I-IV and V (node-negative and node-positive patients) are shown in Figure 1.

Conclusions

This data suggests that clinical trials are the proper context for the study of the impact of familiality on outcome. In early breast cancer patients the outcome of women with and without a family history was similar.

Clinical trials are also adequate for the study of the differences in disease characteristics of patients with and without family history, and they can help identify families with a high cancer occurrence. They are not the correct context for the evaluation of incidence of familiality.

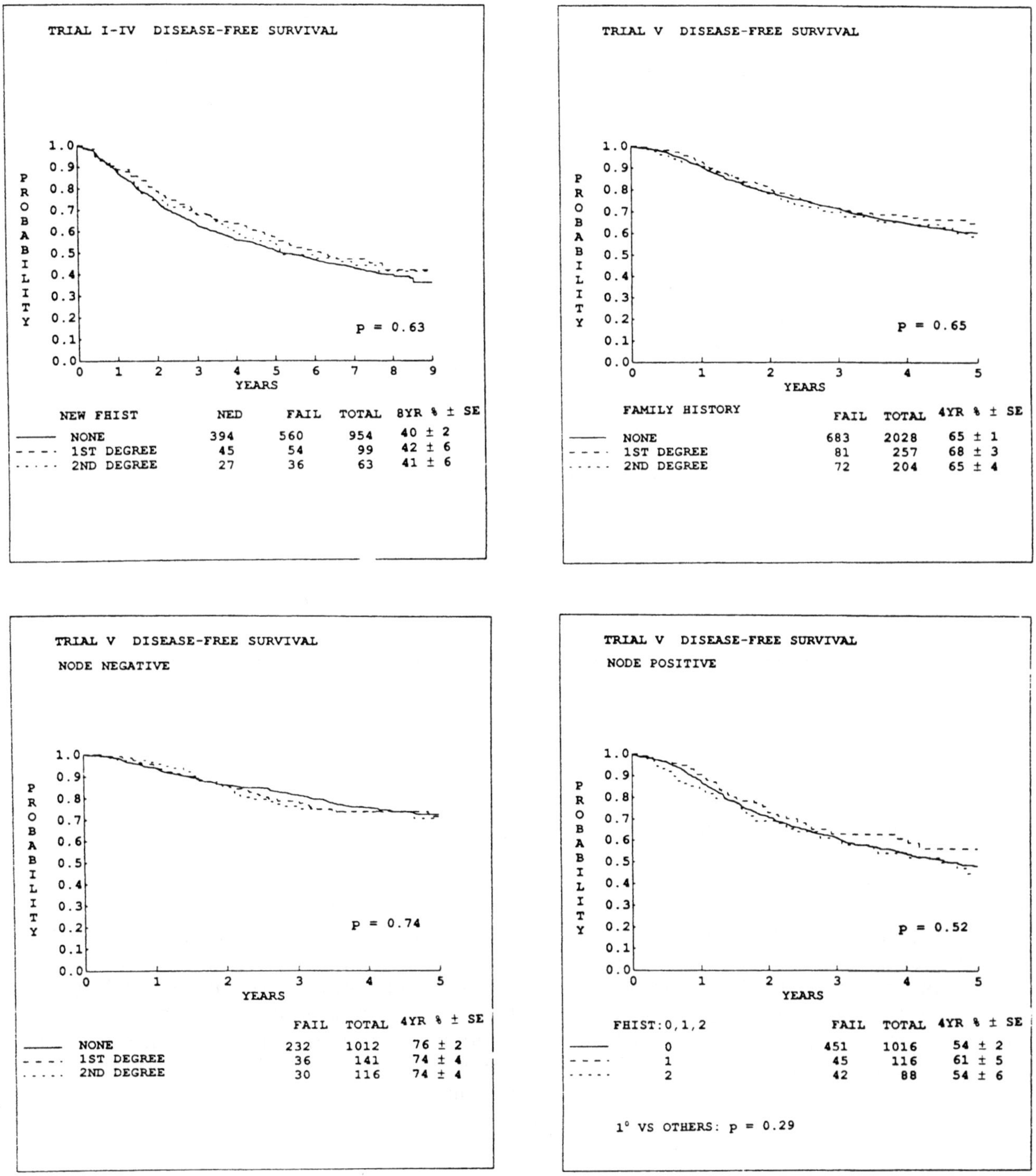

Fig. 1. Disease-free survival curves for studies I-IV and V

Aetiology and Epidemiology - Report of Rapporteur

R.H.Sijmons

Department of Medical Genetics, Faculty of Medicine, University of Groningen, The Netherlands

Gebhardt discussed computerised Markov analysis as a tool to evaluate data on the occurrence of cancer in families registered at the Basel general cancer registry. Using this method in the study of first-degree relatives of probands with colorectal cancer, a higher than expected frequency of this cancer was found, concentrating in the younger age group. Endometrium cancer occurred more frequently than expected in sisters of the probands, but not in their mothers. As was suggested in the discussion, a possible interpretation of this last difference could be the paternal contribution to the transmission of genetic susceptibility to the tumours involved. Computerised Markov analysis could offer hope to those trying to evaluate more complex data in their family studies, as for example the interactions with time-related exogenous factors like smoking.

Scott presented data on Swiss families with adenomatous polyposis coli. A large family was shown in which some members presented with polyposis coli, while in another segment of the family Gardner's syndrome occurred. The two disorders show a great overlap in their clinical picture. Whether or not they should be regarded as separate diseases was discussed with the audience.

Bishop showed the results of a Melbourne study on the occurrence of colorectal cancer among relatives of probands with this disease. Of various genetic models, an autosomal dominant inheritance fits the data best. The postulated gene is associated with risk at early ages of bowel cancer, but is not associated with the other features of HNPCC, suggesting a class of genes different from those thought to be involved in the Lynch syndromes. Mentioned in the discussion was the fact that the Melbourne study has a bias towards left-sided colorectal cancer. Only a small minority of families in this study showed second-degree relatives with colorectal cancer in the absence of first-degree relatives with the disease.

Imam presented a study on a cell surface antigen detected by the anti-NEA 135 antibody in normal mammary epithelial cells, but not in tissue of advanced breast cancer and some other malignant tumours, like colon carcinoma. Early stage breast cancer had not yet been studied. A possible relation between the loss (of detection) of the antigen and chromosome 1p deletions was discussed. The exact nature of this membrane protein and its possible value as a biological marker for the progress of cancer and as a prognostic indicator are still unknown.

Stemmermann discussed the familial occurrence of stomach cancer in Hawaii Japanese. A remarkable finding in this study was the presence of Epstein-Barr virus in a significant proportion of the stomach cancers. A hypothesis was presented in which environmental factors are claimed to be responsible for site selection and actual tumour induction is genetically determined.

Sigg showed the results of several Swiss studies on the familial occurrence of malignant melanomas and dysplastic naevi. Families with dysplastic naevus syndrome showed an excess of stomach cancer. A major problem in studying naevi is that of classification. A general consensus on criteria is urgently needed.

Castiglione presented preliminary data on the value of family history as a prognostic indicator in clinical trials of radically operated breast cancer and colorectal cancer patients. It was concluded from these data that family history had no significant prognostic value in this setting. In the discussion it was emphasised that this conclusion is not valid in the group of families with hereditary breast cancer. A breast-saving operation (lumpectomy) should not be performed in women with hereditary breast cancer; a more radical approach should be taken instead because of the often multifocal and bilateral nature of the disease.

Lynch Syndromes

Lynch Syndromes I and II - Natural History, Diagnosis and Control Strategies

Henry T. Lynch[1], Jane F. Lynch[1] and Giuseppe Cristofaro[2]

1 Department of Preventive Medicine/Public Health, Creighton University School of Medicine, Omaha, Nebraska 68178, U.S.A.

2 Hereditary Gastrointestinal Cancer Prevention Centre, Brindisi, Italy

Hereditary non-polyposis colorectal cancer (HNPCC) is an autosomal dominantly inherited disorder which often shows a distinctive natural history but which lacks any well-defined phenotypic stigmata or biomarkers of cancer susceptibility. This is in striking contrast to its familial adenomatous polyposis (FAP) counterpart, with its distinguishing phenotype of multiple colonic polyps. In addition, the recent identification and characterisation of the APC gene in this region, and demonstration that FAP is caused by mutations in this gene, will enable studies that will define this disease at the biochemical level [1-4]. This discovery adds an entirely new dimension to FAP and may harbour important pathogenetic implications to cancer in general. In comparison to FAP, an HNPCC diagnosis is wholly dependent upon the recognition of certain salient features of its natural history in concert with a detailed pedigree based upon a family history of cancer of *all* anatomic sites.

HNPCC is operationally classified as follows: Lynch syndrome I, which is characterised by an autosomal dominantly inherited susceptibility to colorectal cancer in the absence of multiple colonic polyps, with early age at onset, proclivity to proximal anatomic location, and an excess of synchronous and metachronous colonic cancers; and Lynch syndrome II, which shows all of the features of Lynch syndrome I but, in addition, exhibits a pattern of extracolonic cancers, particularly carcinoma of the endometrium and ovary, which appear to be inherited on the same gene as the colon cancer [5].

Comment

There are more than 200 well-defined hereditary cancer syndromes [5-11]. This listing will undoubtedly increase as clinicians devote greater attention to the cancer family history and, concurrently, as molecular genetic advances provide new clues about the existence of cancer genes. Security in hereditary cancer syndrome diagnosis will be enhanced commensurate with research devoted to the various clinical and pathological aspects of the phenotype(s). The gold standard for precision in hereditary cancer syndrome identification will rest on a meticulously defined phenotype in context with molecular genetic correlation of genotypic susceptibility to cancer.

Genetic cancer diagnosis is relatively easy and straightforward in the more than 50 cancer-associated genodermatoses [8]. In these settings, cutaneous signs will provide important clues to the underlying hereditary syndrome. However, in the case of the Lynch syndromes, with the exception of cutaneous signs of the Muir-Torre syndrome, namely, multiple sebaceous adenomas, sebaceous carcinomas, and/or keratoacanthomas in rare examples of Lynch syndrome II [12,13], no such phenotypic stigmata are present and to date there are no consistent biomarkers of acceptable sensitivity and specificity to its cancer-prone genotype(s). Evidence indicating the location of the susceptibility locus remains elusive. For example, the Kidd blood group locus on chromosome 18 had been considered as a candidate site for the Lynch syndrome II gene [14], but recent work by

Peltomaki et al. [15] has suggested that this region is not the site of the subject gene. It is for this reason that the clinician must rely fully on the mentioned features of the Lynch syndromes' natural history, inclusive of tumour spectrum and family history, with an extended pedigree, all in context with knowledge of hereditary cancer's differential diagnosis.

Differential Diagnosis of the Lynch Syndromes

The clinician must make a distinction between HNPCC and other hereditary colorectal cancer counterparts, particularly the several FAP syndromes [5,16]. The exclusion of FAP syndromes can often be made through recognition of multiple (particularly florid) colonic polyps or, in the case of the so-called Gardner's variant, in addition to colonic polyposis, the presence of extracolonic signs such as osteomas, cutaneous cysts, desmoid tumours [17] and congenital hypertrophy of the retinal pigment epithelium (CHRPE) [18].
One must also consider problems of heterogeneity in the FAP syndromes, including variable expressivity of the colonic adenomatous polyp phenotype [19], findings which could be confused with HNPCC. Consideration must also be given to hereditary isolated common polyp-colon cancer-prone families as described by Burt et al. [20] and Cannon-Albright et al. [21]. This disorder may be difficult to distinguish from HNPCC and, to a lesser extent, the FAP syndromes. Significant extension of the pedigree will be important in deriving these distinctions.
The recently described hereditary flat adenoma syndrome (HFAS) must also enter into this differential diagnosis [22,23]. HFAS is characterised by an autosomal dominant inheritance pattern which predisposes patients to flat adenomas (FAs), with proximal colonic predominance, fundic gland polyps, and colorectal cancer which has a later age of onset than that found in FAP and HNPCC but which is earlier than that found in so-called sporadic colorectal cancer. HFAS is linked to the FAP susceptibility locus on chromosome 5 [23].
HNPCC must also be distinguished from familial colorectal cancer (two or more first- or second-degree relatives with colorectal cancer). When considering familial aggregation as well as sporadic occurrences of colorectal cancer, one must realise how common colorectal cancer is in the general population, particularly in western industrialised nations [24]. Hence, multiple colorectal cancer case families will be encountered frequently on the basis of chance alone. It is clear that the differentiation of all forms of familial or hereditary clusters of colorectal cancer from HNPCC will require attention to natural history, age at onset, multiple primary cancer, and site predilection within the colon [5].

Tumour Spectrum in HNPCC

The frequency of specific types of cancer has been recently analysed in members of 23 HNPCC families from the Creighton University/Hereditary Cancer Institute resource [25]. We compared the observed numbers of cancer diagnoses in each risk group to the expected numbers, based on general population incidence data.
Members of this high-risk group had significantly ($p<0.05$) more cancer diagnoses at specific sites than expected. Sites where cancer was found to occur in excess included stomach, small intestine, hepatobiliary system, kidney/ureter, and ovary. Colorectal and endometrial cancers were not studied since they were used in the risk group classification. No differences were found between males and females in the cohort, except for the excess of ovarian cancer.
No excess of pancreatic cancer, lymphatic/haematopoietic cancer, laryngeal cancer, breast cancer, malignant brain tumours, or lung/bronchus cancer was detected in the high-risk group. In fact, significantly *fewer* lung/bronchus cancer cases occurred than were expected ($p<0.05$). None of the 5 reported cases occurred in the affected or unaffected gene carriers.
Anecdotal occurrences of carcinoma of the pancreas, however, have been observed in Lynch syndrome II kindreds [26,27]. In one such family, 3 relatives in the direct genetic lineage manifested carcinoma of the pancreas.
Lynch et al. [28] observed biliary tract and duodenum cancer in 2 members of an HNPCC kindred. Of interest is the fact that

biliary and ampullary tumours are common in patients with FAP [29-31]. Preoperative gastroscopy and abdominal ultrasonography prior to colorectal surgery is therefore indicated for those patients with Lynch syndrome II wherein these lesions have been observed in the family. Needle cholangiography would be indicated in the presence of biliary tract abnormalities. Liver function studies would also be appropriate.

Vasen et al. [32] studied the tumour complement in 24 HNPCC kindreds from Holland. Colorectal cancer was present in 104 patients, where the mean age at diagnosis was 46 years. In 4 of the families, colorectal cancer was the only type of cancer to occur, a finding consonant with the Lynch symdrome I variant. Sixty-five extracolonic tumours were observed in 20 of the kindreds. Carcinoma of the endometrium was present in 16 patients from 12 families; carcinoma of the stomach was present in 10 patients from 5 families, primarily in the older generations; and urinary tract tumours were found in 8 patients from 4 families. Other forms of cancer were observed but at a lesser frequency. These investigators concluded that carcinoma of the endometrium, stomach, and urinary tract were integral to the hereditary tumour spectrum of HNPCC.

Future studies of the tumour spectrum in HNPCC should focus on several important tasks. Firstly, additional data on cancer diagnoses with exact descriptions of site and histology, should be accumulated. This is especially important in complex systems such as the hepatic/biliary/pancreatic system.

Secondly, larger data bases or meta-analysis should be used to evaluate more subtle differences between cancer in HNPCC family members and its occurrence in the general population.

Finally, the issue of heterogeneity must be addressed. Are there differences between HNPCC families in the risk for endometrial, urological, or other extracolonic cancers? If so, these differences might reflect a fundamental difference in the underlying inherited disorder. One sort of heterogeneity has been hypothesised: Lynch syndrome I vs. Lynch syndrome II, as described above. It is also possible that other special subtypes could be identified, based on the family history of cancer at specific organ sites occurring in conjunction with colorectal cancer. Analyses testing specific hypotheses about heterogeneity will facilitate development of cancer control programmes, allow more sophisticated genetic studies, and clarify concepts and hypotheses about possible mechanisms of cancer susceptibility in HNPCC.

Screening - Management of High-Risk Family Members

The consistency of the natural history features seen in HNPCC, such as proximal colon predilection, synchronous and metachronous colorectal cancer, and the pattern of associated cancers of specific targeted organs, has immediate pertinence to the development of surveillance and management strategies for these families. For example, in all of the kindreds, colonoscopy is mandated. If we employed the alternative of flexible sigmoidoscopic examination, we would miss more than two-thirds of the cancers, given the predilection for the proximal colon. If the surgeon performed a limited colorectal cancer resection, such as a hemicolectomy, the patient would remain vulnerable for metachronous cancer involving the remaining colonic segment. Hence, subtotal colectomy is necessary. Women in the direct genetic lineage who have completed their families and who present with colorectal cancer, should become candidates for prophylactic total abdominal hysterectomy-bilateral salpingo-oophorectomy (TAH-BSO) because of their inordinately increased risk for carcinoma of the endometrium and ovary.

Screening strategies necessarily must initiate much *earlier* in life because of the early onset aspect of cancer's natural history in the Lynch syndromes. Depending on the age of onset of colorectal cancer in a given family, we initiate colonoscopy between ages 20-25. This must be repeated every other year through age 35, and then annually thereafter. There is no age at which we can safely state that the patient is no longer at risk for colorectal cancer. In addition, as the patient's age increases, the cancer risk also increases in accord with the population risk for colorectal cancer, which is age dependent. Therefore, we believe it prudent to continue colonoscopic screening for the rest of the patient's life. With respect to gynaecologic cancer, we recommend initiation of endometrial aspiration biopsy and transvaginal ultrasound, along with CA-125, beginning at age 25 and annually for the rest of the patient's life.

Summary and Conclusions

In summary, knowledge of family history and the natural history of the cancer phenotype provides a powerful basis for diagnosis, surveillance and management. In Lynch syndrome I, the primary surveillance and management focus is on the colorectum. In Lynch syndrome II, these strategies are more complex because of the excess risk for extracolonic cancer. Differentiation of these syndromes is also essential for investigation of genetic/environmental interaction in their aetiology as well as for the development of strategies for biomarker investigations. Given the advances in molecular genetics during the past decade, attention must now be focused appropriately upon the search for identification of the responsible gene(s) in HNPCC through the help of recombinant DNA techniques [33]. Experience from the FAP model [1-4,34] may one day be applied to the Lynch syndromes. This research will undoubtedly facilitate improvement in HNPCC's surveillance and management strategies. However, central to this entire project is the need to integrate the natural history of the Lynch syndrome phenotype into any newly developing strategies for diagnosis, surveillance and management.

REFERENCES

1 Groden J, Thliveris A, Samowitz W et al: Identification and characterization of the familial adenomatous polyposis coli gene. Cell 1991 (66):589-600

2 Joslyn G, Carlson M, Thliveris A et al: Identification of deletion mutations and three new genes at the familial polyposis locus. Cell 1991 (66):601-613

3 Kinzler KW, Nilbert MC, Su LK et al: Identification of FAP locus genes from chromosome 5q21. Science 1991 (253):661-665

4 Nishisho I, Nakamura Y, Mioshi Y et al: Mutations of chromosome 5q21 genes in FAP and colorectal cancer patients. Science 1991 (253):665-669

5 Lynch PM and Lynch HT: Colon Cancer Genetics. VN Reinhold, New York 1985

6 Lynch HT: Cancer Genetics. CC Thomas, Springfield 1976

7 Lynch HT: Genetics and Breast Cancer. VN Reinhold, New York 1981

8 Lynch HT and Fusaro RM: Cancer-Associated Genodermatoses. VN Reinhold, New York 1981

9 Lynch HT and Kullander S: Cancer Genetics in Women. CRC Press, Boca Raton 1987

10 Lynch HT and Hirayama T: Genetic Epidemiology of Cancer. CRC Press, Boca Raton 1989

11 Utsunomiya J and Lynch HT: Hereditary colorectal Cancer. Springer Verlag, Tokyo 1990

12 Lynch HT, Lynch PM, Pester J and Fusaro RM: The cancer family syndrome: rare cutaneous phenotypic linkage of Torre's syndrome. Arch Int Med 1980 (141):607-611

13 Lynch HT, Fusaro RM, Roberts L, Voorhees GJ and Lynch JF: Muir-Torre syndrome in several members of a family with a variant of the Cancer Family Syndrome. Br J Dermatol 1985 (113):295-301

14 Lynch HT, Kimberling WJ, Albano W et al: Hereditary nonpolyposis colorectal cancer (Lynch syndromes I and II). Cancer 1985 (56):939-951

15 Peltomaki P, Sistonen P, Mecklin J-P et al: Evidence supporting exclusion of the DCC gene and a portion of chromosome 18q as the locus for susceptibility to hereditary nonpolyposis colorectal carcinoma in five kindreds. Cancer Res 1991 (51):4135-4140

16 Lynch HT, Watson P, Kriegler M et al: Differential diagnosis of hereditary nonpolyposis colorectal cancer (Lynch syndrome I and Lynch syndrome II). Dis Colon Rect 1988 (31):372-377

17 Jagelman DG: Extracolonic manifestations of familial polyposis coli. Cancer Genet Cytogenet 1987 (31):372-377

18 Traboulsi EI, Krush AJ, Gardner EJ et al: Prevalence and importance of pigmented ocular fundus lesions in Gardner's syndrome. N Engl J Med 1987 (316):661-667

19 Lynch HT, Lynch PM, Follett KL and Harris RE: Familial polyposis coli: heterogeneous polyp expression in two kindreds. J Med Genet 1979 (16):1-7

20 Burt RW, Bishop DT, Cannon LA, Dowdle MA, Lee RG and Skolnick MH: Dominant inheritance of adenomatous colonic polyps and colorectal cancer. N Engl J Med 1985 (312):1540-1544

21 Cannon-Albright LA, Skolnick MH, Bishop DJ et al: Common inheritance of susceptibility to colonic adenomatous polyps and associated colorectal cancer. N Engl J Med 1988 (319):533-537

22 Lynch HT, Smyrk T, Lanspa SJ et al: Flat adenomas in a colon cancer-prone kindred. JNCI 1988 (80):278-282

23 Lynch HT, Smyrk TC, Lanspa SJ et al: Phenotypic variation in colorectal adenoma/cancer expression in two families: hereditary flat adenoma syndrome. Cancer 1990 (66):909-915

24 Boring CC, Squires TS, Tong T: Cancer statistics, 1991. Cancer 1991 (41):19-51

25 Watson P and Lynch HT: Extracolonic cancer in HNPCC: application to linkage analysis. In: Proc of the 4th International Symposium on Colorectal Cancer. Springer Verlag, Tokyo 1990 pp 119-126

26 Lynch HT, Voorhees GJ, Lanspa SJ et al: Pancreatic carcinoma and hereditary nonpolyposis colorectal cancer: a family study. Br J Cancer 1985 (52):271-273

27 Lynch HT, Smyrk TC, Lynch PM et al: Adenocarcinoma of the small bowell in Lynch syndrome II. Cancer 1989 (64):2178-2183

28 Jagelman DG, DeCosse JJ and Bussey HJR: Upper gastrointestinal cancer in familial adenomatous polyposis. Lancet 1989 (i):1149-1151

29 Jarvinen HF and Sipponen P: Gastroduodenal polyps in familial adenomatous and juvenile polyposis. Endoscopy 1986 (18):230-234

30 Lynch HT, Fitzsimmons ML, Smyrk TC et al: Familial pancreatic cancer: clinicopathologic study of 18 nuclear families. Am J Gastroent 1990 (85):54-60

31 Sugihara K, Muto T, Kamiya J et al: Gardner syndrome associated with periampullary carcinoma, duodenal and gastric adenomatosis. Dis Colon Rect 1982 (25):766-771

32 Vasen HFA, Offerhaus GJA, den Hartog Jager et al: The tumor spectrum in hereditary nonpolyposis colorectal cancer: a study of 24 kindreds in the Netherlands. Int J Cancer 1990 (46):31-34

33 Nakamura Y, White R, Smitts AMM and Bos JL: Genetic alterations during colorectal-tumor development. N Engl J Med 1988 (319):525-532

34 Petersen GM, Slack J and Nakamura Y: Screening guidelines for at risk relatives of familial adenomatous polyposis (FAP) with genetic linkage data. Gastroenterology 1990 (98):A303 (abstract)

Cost-Benefit Implications in the Surveillance of Lynch Syndrome Subjects

Giuseppe Cristofaro[1], Eupremio Carrozzo [2], Frederick Gentile [3] and Emilio Di Giulio [4]

1 Hereditary Gastrointestinal Cancer Prevention Centre, Brindisi, Italy
2 Head of the Statistics Office, Chamber of Commerce, Brindisi, Italy
3 British Consulate, Brindisi, Italy
4 Vth Surgical Clinic, Department of Endoscopy, "La Sapienza" University, Rome, Italy

Hereditary diseases, especially tumours of the gastrointestinal (GI) tract, are gaining interest throughout the world [1,2]. They represent a unique model for the understanding of the aetiology of cancer and its biological behaviour, enabling us to introduce preventive strategies and possibly newer, more sophisticated therapies which are currently being searched for by molecular biologists [3].

Among hereditary precancerous conditions, familial adenomatous polyposis (FAP), and its variant, the Gardner Syndrome (GS), were, until a few years ago, the most recognised and investigated. Another condition at very high risk for GI cancer is being a first-degree relative in a family showing the Lynch syndromes, recently called *Hereditary Non-Polyposis Colorectal Cancer* (HNPCC). Subjects prone to FAP (GS) or HNPCC develop the disease when they are young, i.e., starting at or during the fully productive age. Since the disease is characterised by dominant transmission, 50% of descendants in a family in which HNPCC occurs develop cancer.

The main differences between FAP or GS and HNPCC are: a) a significant lack of polyps in HNPCC compared to FAP in which more than 500 polyps are spread on all colonic segments; b) FAP represents about 1% of the colon cancer burden as opposed to more than 6% as accurately estimated for HNPCC [4,5]; c) the third, possibly most important difference, in terms of public or private assistance and cost implications, lies in the fact that 1) FAP polyps are truly precancerous *lesions* and as such recognised as true disease; 2) HNPCC is a serious precancerous *condition*, given the absence, at least at present, of instrumentally demonstrable lesions.

This last, crucial point represents the most important medical problem regarding early detection of GI cancer in Lynch syndromes. It becomes, therefore, fundamental to identify families showing peculiarities suggesting HNPCC by means of a more in-depth investigation of cancer family history in subjects with colon cancer or right-sided adenomas, especially diminutive adenomas, when detected under the age of 50.

Such anamnetic accuracy is the first and main requirement for offering young subjects with HNPCC a normal working life *before* or *after cancer*, by entrusting them to *specialised* centres that are equipped for a better management of their health.

The benefit society could achieve by financing these specialised centres is the main topic of this paper. Our intention was to examine the above situation in terms of its implications for society from the point of view of cost and productivity as well as to demonstrate what the impact of secondary prevention on young subjects showing Lynch syndromes would be in economic terms. This analysis also attempts to provide a "common ground" on which the needs of medical ethics and the demands and constraints of today's cost-conscious society can perhaps meet.

Methods

The Italian health care system has been taken as an example, with special emphasis on assistance costs versus benefits achieved. The following criteria were taken into account:

a) HNPCC incidence (for colon and stomach only);
b) Yearly expenses made by a specialised centre in managing these subjects;
c) For an easier understanding, the costs per year of instrumental examinations in the management of Italian subjects were estimated and added;
d) Subject compliance rate;
e) Average age at cancer death in HNPCC (for colon and gastric localisations only);
f) Returns to society on the basis of productive capacity expressed in monetary terms. This value has been calculated as follows:
   Gross Domestic Product (GDP) .... A
   divided by
   No. of economically active population
   (age group 20-60) .... B
   Productive capacity of each
   working individual .... Z

Although Z could suffice as a *prima facie* indicator, we feel that a more realistic figure is obtained by subtracting the operating costs (C) involved in achieving the Gross Domestic Product, namely, indirect taxes net of subsidies and employee compensation. The result of this calculation (Y) is the net operating surplus, i.e., the amount a person produces in real terms net of all costs, hence:

$$Z - C = Y$$

(where Y = GDP per capita of the economically active population less operating costs).

From this figure we can see how important, in financial terms, a subject aged between 20 and 60 years is to society or, in other words, what society will lose if a young subject is struck by cancer during his working life.
According to an adapted version of the instrumental guidelines developed by the International Collaborative Group on HNPCC, Italian subjects at high risk should undergo a colonoscopy every 2 years in the age group 25-35, and once yearly in the age group 35-60. In families where gastric cancer represents more than 10% of all cancers, a gastroscopy is also recommended with the same time intervals as those mentioned above.
Data regarding colon and gastric cancer incidence has been provided by the Epidemiological Service of the National Cancer Institute of Italy. Gastric cancer incidence in HNPCC has been conservatively estimated at 10% of all HNPCC cases. Statistics regarding the potential value in terms of benefits have been provided by the Central Institute of Statistics (Italy). The mean currency of U.S.$ for 1991 has been furnished by the Italian Central Exchange Office.

Results

The incidence of gastrointestinal cancer, in particular located in the colon and stomach, is reported in Table 1.
Table 2 summarises the costs.
Average age at cancer death is shown in Table 3.
Real productive capacity per year in financial terms of each working individual aged 20-60, is summarised in Table 4.
Table 5 summarises the annual financial difference between the costs of subject management compared to net productive capacity of each working individual.
The compliance of subjects to undergo secondary prevention was 89% in the Apulia region (Italy), according to the Hereditary Gastrointestinal Cancer Prevention Centre of Brindisi, Italy.

Discussion

From the figures shown in Table 4 it can be seen that the real productive capacity in monetary terms in Italy is equal to U.S. $ 31,153 per individual. If we consider that, in general, 50% of GI cancer-prone subjects develop the disease we can surmise that, in the case of Italian subjects affected by HNPCC, lives lost could be estimated to be about 400 (800 x 50%) per year, which means that the economy is deprived of a sum of almost U.S. $ 12,461,200 per annum.
If we then take into account that the average age of death for HNPCC subjects with colon cancer, 369 in Italy (738 x 50%), is 39, and that the working life expectancy is a further 20 years, it can be argued that the economy sustains, in theory, a loss of approximately

Table 1. Incidence of gastrointestinal cancer in Italy

Population	GI cancer incidence		HNPCC incidence = 6%	
	Colon	**Stomach**		
57,739,247	21.3/100,000 = 12,298	23.6/100,000 = 13,626	**Colon = 738**	**Stomach (10%) = 74**

data refer to 1990

Table 2. Cost summary related to Italy

Centre management/year		$ 140,000
Colonoscopy/each*	$ 1,350 x 738	$ 996,300
Gastroscopy *	$ 430 x 74	$ 31,820
Total costs per year		$ 1,168,120

* based on commercial costs for private treatment in 1990

Table 3. Average age at death in HNPCC subjects

Colon	39	Stomach	42

Table 4. Real productive capacity for working individuals aged 20-60 in Italy

(A)	Gross Domestic Product (G.D.P.)	$ 1,078,236,566,534
(B)	Economically active population (age 20-60)	# 19,297,000
(Z)	G.D.P. pro capita of economically active population	$ 55,876
(C)	Operating costs pro capita	$ 24,723
(Y)	Net productive capacity of each working individual	$ 31,153

data refer to 1990

Table 5. Difference between costs of subject management and net productive capacity in Italy

Colonoscopy cost per subject, per year	$	1,350*
Gastroscopy cost per subject, per year	$	430*
Management costs (centres) per subject, per year	$	172
(X) Total costs per subject, per year	$	1,952**
(Y) Net productive capacity of each working individual	$	31,153
Balance (Y-X)	**$**	**29,201**

* private costs (not common in Italy by virtue of free, public assistance)
** costs altered by private costs of instrumental examinations
Data refer to 1990

U.S. $ 229,909,140 over that period. This estimate, however, is based on 369 lives, i.e., victims claimed in 1 year, and does not take into account growth and inflation factors. In reality, the final figure is enormous.
A glance at Table 5 shows the cost of managing a subject, his/her net productive capacity and the difference between the two. It is obvious from the difference that the benefits achieved by providing *preventive medicine* and thus saving a life outweigh the costs of doing so by a staggering $ 29,201 per subject, per year (in Italy). We believe that this is also a conservative estimate because for technical reasons we are not able to calculate costs incurred for hospitalisation, drugs, and treatment before the subject died. It is easy to understand that such costs in many cases can be extremely high and to very little avail. At this point, we would suggest that the "cost" of supervising a subject at risk should be taken as an *investment*, especially when one considers that the return is over 15 times the original figure.

Conclusions

The statistics summarised here show the invaluable importance of secondary prevention in terms of cost savings and returns that can be achieved by a society prepared to make the investments necessary for such strategies.
Due to the early age at onset of cancer seen in the Lynch syndromes and to the fact that subjects greatly outnumber FAP cases (6 times as many), prevention procedures organised by specialised centres for subjects prone to these syndromes are not simply another burden on public health budgets, but a real investment with a tangible return.
Contrary to what is seen in most countries where the health care system is privatised, i.e., primarily based on private medical insurance, Italy offers indiscriminate medical protection to all citizens who comply with preventive screening. In other countries, and particularly in the U.S.A., the insurance covers only the costs of therapy and diagnosis when the patient falls ill. Insurance policies do not cover routine screening procedures aimed at preventing a certain disease; the costs thereof have to be paid by the individual. This work demonstrates that in HNPCC patients more consideration should be given to this particular disease because the economic advantages society obtains are much greater than the costs of managing these subjects. Free, government-funded examinations could also improve the compliance rate, as can be seen in Italy. Paradoxically, the higher the complicance, and thus the costs, the greater the economic benefits achieved by society.
Given the current climate of the world economy, we consider it appropriate to deal with the problem both in general terms, i.e., considering the effective cost to society for secondary prevention and the benefits that it would yield, and in specific terms, i.e., considering the numerous cases handled by specialised centres and the *restitutio ad integrum* of young lives that are substantially below the pensionable age with a subsequent recovery in the productive economy.
Clearly, the methods described in this paper refer to summary statistics reported with an outline interpretation. They are, however, not intended to be definitive but should constitute a "starting point" for further analysis and discussion, hopefully involving personnel specialised in the field of social economics and ideally in collaboration with their medical counterparts.
We would conclude by saying that it is not at all banal to emphasise the term *investment* if one considers the cost-benefit ratio and the economic advantages that productive society could obtain from *specific* and *targeted* cancer screening in fighting this oncological phenomenon, provided that such prevention strategies are managed and scheduled by specialised centres.
We feel, however, that it is of the utmost importance to point out that in any approach to medicine the paramount factor must always remain that of saving lives and eliminating disease. As we said in our introduction, the aim of this paper is to preserve the integrity of medical ethics but, at the same time, establish compatibility with the economic goals and restrictions of an ever developing society.

REFERENCES

1 Lynch HT, Lanspa SJ, Smyrk TC, Fitzgibbons RJ, Watson P, Boman BM, Lynch JF and Cristofaro G: Historical and natural cancer history facets of the Lynch Syndromes. In: Utsunomiya J and Lynch HT (eds) Hereditary Colon Cancer. Springer Verlag, Tokyo, Berlin, Heidelberg, New York, London, Paris, Hong Kong, Barcelona 1990 pp 17-25

2 Cristofaro G, Lynch HT, Caruso ML, Attolini A et al: New phenotypic aspects in a family with Lynch Syndrome II. Cancer 1987 (60):51-58

3 Vogelstein B, Fearon ER, Hamilton SR, Bodmer WF, Jass JR, Jeffreys AJ, Lucibello FC, Patel I and Rider SH: Genetic alterations during colorectal tumor development. N Engl J Med 1988 (319):525-532

4 Lynch HT: Frequency of hereditary nonpolyposis colorectal cancer. Gastroenterology 1986 (90):486-492

5 Mecklin JP: Frequency of hereditary colorectal cancer. Gastroenterology 1987 (93):1021-1025

Treatment

Is Endoscopy Still Controversial in Secondary Prevention of Colon Cancer?

Rémy Meier and Klaus Gyr

Department of Internal Medicine, Gastroenterology, Kantonsspital Liestal and University of Basel, Switzerland

Colorectal cancer (CRC) is one of the leading causes of death from cancer in most industrialised countries. In Switzerland there are about 4000 new cases and 2000 deaths per year. The overall risk of having CRC by the age of 75 is approximately 3.5%. The natural history of CRC offers several opportunities for intervention. It is widely accepted that in most cases, CRC progresses from normal colonic mucosa to benign adenomatous polyps, to early curable tumours, and finally to advanced and incurable cancer [1-3]. The estimated time course of this evolution is about 10 to 15 years. Screening procedures should be able to intervene in this fatal sequence. CRC is a prime target for screening because it is a major health problem, the disease remains in a detectable and early preclinical phase for a long time, and early treatment by surgical resection or endoscopic eradication of adenomatous polyps improves survival rates. Five screening methods aimed at detecting premalignant or early stages of carcinoma are discussed, and the value of each test is briefly considered.

Screening Procedures

The screening tests currently recommended are digital rectal examination, the faecal occult blood test, sigmoidoscopy, barium air contrast enema and colonoscopy, alone or in combination. None of these tests has been shown to have the ideal characteristics of being highly effective, acceptable, easy to perform, non-invasive and cheap. All screening procedures are debatable, because none of these tests has yet been shown to produce a real reduction of mortality.

Digital rectal examination is a cheap and well tolerated examination. However, only 10% of all tumours can be reached by palpation [4].

Faecal occult blood test: This test, based on a guaiac-basis, is the most widely applied screening test with a compliance rate of 50 to 75% [5-7]. In order to test its effectiveness in detecting early stages of CRC, 5 large studies were initiated. The rate of positive tests in the screened population was 1-2.4% (non-hydrated slides). The predictive value for detecting adenomas or carcinomas in those patients with positive faecal occult blood test results, who were further examined, was between 30 and 58%. In all screened patients, the proportion of Duke's A and B tumours was higher than in the control group (65-90% vs 33-55%) [8-12]. Faecal occult blood tests are easy to perform, cheap and have no adverse effects. Drawbacks are false-positive rates of 1-5%, leading to unnecessary and expensive diagnostic evaluation and high false-negative rates (35-50%) due to bleeding being intermittent or to blood loss being slight. No reduction of mortality has been reported up to now [5].

Sigmoidoscopy: The effectiveness of sigmoidoscopy for screening is not well evaluated. The proportion of detectable tumours lies between 30 and 50% with rigid and 60% with flexible sigmoidoscopy. Due to the tendency of colon cancer to be on the right side, a considerable number of colonic neoplasms (25-45%) will be missed. Two large uncontrolled studies and 1 randomised controlled study with rigid sigmoidoscopy showed no real decrease in cancer mortality [13-16]. For flexible sigmoidoscopy, no controlled trials, either completed or in progress, are available.

Air contrast barium enema and colonoscopy are well accepted methods for examining the entire colon. Both procedures have a high detection rate for neoplasms (90-95%). When the 2 methods are compared, the air contrast barium enema is less sensitive than colonoscopy [17-19]. For several reasons, colonoscopy is attractive for screening because of the high detection rate even for small lesions, the low false-positive rate and the possibility of taking biopsy samples or performing polypectomy. The main disadvantages are the high cost and the risks of perforation (0.2-0.4%) and bleeding (0.7-2.5%), mainly due to polypectomy.

Screening by Endoscopy

Colonoscopy has high costs and work load, and a risk of complications. Nevertheless, it is the screening method with the highest detection rate for colorectal malignancy, and its use offers the possibility of intervening directly in the adenoma-carcinoma sequence.

Therefore, it seems reasonable to screen persons at high risk of developing colorectal malignancy by colonoscopy. High-risk persons are defined by having a positive family history and being over 50 years old (Table 1).

Table 1. Risk groups for CRC screening

High risk

Positive family history

- Rare hereditary syndromes
  - Polyposis syndromes
  - HNPCC (Lynch I and II)
- First-degree relatives of patients with sporadic colon cancer
- First-degree relatives of patients with adenomas

Average risk

Men and women 50 years of age and older

There is general agreement that screening patients with familial polyposis syndromes and their relatives by procto-sigmoidoscopy-colonoscopy reduces the risk for CRC when screening is started at the age of 10 to 12 years. Colonoscopy is not necessary all the time, because the polyps occur in the whole colon. When polyps occur, colectomy has to be planned.

First-degree relatives of patients with hereditary non-polyposis colon cancer (HNPCC), also known as Lynch syndrome I/II, have an up to 8-fold increased risk of CRC [20, 21]. For this group it is becoming apparent that colonoscopy is the screening method of choice because of the high risk and the predominance of the cancer localised in the proximal colon. Screening should begin 5 to 10 years before the first cancer has appeared in the family. The cost and work load are acceptable in this relatively small group, because only about 6% of all CRCs are hereditary. Long-term and outcome data for such screening programmes are not available.

The largest group of CRC are the sporadic colonic cancers (94%). Several studies have shown at least a 3-fold increase in risk of carcinoma and adenomas in the first-degree relatives [22-28]. Family studies showed an increased risk depending on the number of affected relatives [29]. Five colonoscopic studies in asymptomatic first-degree relatives with a mean age of 53 years (range 23 to 90 years) were performed (Table 2) [30-34]. In a total of 490 subjects, 149 adenomas or carcinomas were found with a range in the different studies of 18 to 63%. In one-third of the adenomas, the lesions were hyperplastic polyps. The importance of these hyperplastic polyps has still not been defined, but it is widely accepted that they do not grow and do not turn into malignant polyps. From the 93 real adenomas, only 15% were villous. A carcinoma was found in less than 1%. Three of these carcinoma patients were older than 60 years and one was 47 years old. On the basis of these data, it is not possible to recommend colonoscopy for mass screening of first-degree relatives in patients with sporadic CRC until more data on cost/effectiveness and a reduction in mortality resulting from such screening programmes have been reported. But we recommend for individual patients that the indications for colonoscopy

Table 2. Screening asymptomatic first-degree relatives with a positive family history for CRC

Author	[ref]	N	Mean age (range)	Adenoma/ Carcinoma N	(%)	Hyper-plastic polyps	Tubular adenoma	Villous adenoma	Carcinoma	% beyond splenic flexure
Gryska	[30]	49	54 (23-81)	31	(63)	12	9	8	2	41
Guillem	[31]	48	55 (32-81)	12	(25)	-	12	-	-	33
Grossmann	[32]	154	54 (30-85)	28	(18)	-	27	1	-	45
Orrom	[33]	114	51 (24-86)	39*	(34)	10	19	2	2	25
McConnell	[35]	125	56 (35-85)	39	(30)	24	15**		-	40
Total		**490**	**53**	**149**	**(30)**	**46**	93		4	

* In 6 no histology was available
** No differentiation between tubular and villous adenoma

should be handled liberally. A decision as to whether screening approaches with colonoscopy for subjects with more complex family histories are more effective must await the results of prospective randomised trials comparing long-term overall and cancer-specific mortality in the screened group with that of the unscreened controls.

First-degree relatives of adenoma patients also have an increased risk for adenomas. Adenomas are very common and the prevalence and size increase with age [35]. Screening first-degree relatives of patients with adenomas may be very attractive because of the possible common inheritance of adenomas and CRC shown by Burt et al. [26] and Cannon et al. [27], but unfortunately the value of this procedure has not yet been established.

There is a lively discussion about the screening by colonoscopy of persons in the average-risk group who are over 45 or 50 years old. The incidence and mortality in men and women sharply increase between 50 and 60 years [35]. However, this is a very large population group to screen (e.g., more than one million inhabitants in Switzerland are over 65 years old). The American National Cancer Institute and the American Cancer Society recommend annual rectal examination and faecal occult blood tests for people over the age of 50 years, and a sigmoidoscopy every 3 to 5 years. However, sigmoidoscopy and faecal occult blood test have not shown a decrease in morbidity and mortality and, furthermore, it has been shown that sigmoidoscopy fails to detect 25 to 45% of neoplasms (Table 2). In the only available study on the use of colonoscopy in the screening of asymptomatic persons over the age of 50, Rex et al. screened 210 such persons with a negative faecal occult blood test. In 53 subjects, adenomas were found and in 2 patients a carcinoma. Eighteen of the 53 lesions were hyperplastic polyps and 35 were adenomas. All patients with an adenoma greater than 1 cm or a carcinoma were over 60 years old [36]. The yield of screening by colonoscopy was, therefore, low in persons aged under 60 years. But over the age of 60, a higher detection rate was demonstrated. From this study we may suggest that it can be recommended that screening by colonoscopy could be started later than at the age of 50 years.

In summary, we conclude that the "gold standard" for screening would be colonoscopy because of the high detection rate of colorectal malignancy and the possibility of intervening in the adenoma-carcinoma sequence.

However, in average-risk persons colonoscopy cannot at present be recommended for mass screening. It has high costs and involves a heavy work load. As yet, there is no direct evidence showing a reduction of mortality when the procedure is used, and safety and cost/effectiveness need to be evaluated in more detail [35]. At the moment, colonoscopy can be recommended in patients and relatives with family polyposis coli syndromes and in relatives of patients with hereditary non-polyposis colonic cancer (HNPCC), or in families with complex family histories. For the near future, we must make every effort to identify either groups with higher risks (e.g., 10-20%) or those with a very low risk (e.g., less than 1%). Maybe genetic markers or complex family histories will help us to identify such groups for screening by colonoscopy or for elimination from screening programmes.

REFERENCES

1 Hill MJ, Morrison BC and Bussey HJR: Aetiology of adenoma-carcinoma sequence in the large bowel. Lancet 1978 (1):245-247

2 Waye JD: Colon polyps: problems, promises, prospects. Am J Gastroenterol 1986 (81):101-103

3 Day DW and Morson BC: The adenoma-carcinoma sequence. In: Morson BC (ed) The Pathogenesis of Colorectal Cancer. WB Saunders, Philadelphia 1978 pp 58-71

4 Winawer SJ: Screening for colorectal cancer. In: De Vita VT, Hellman S, Rosenberg SA (eds) Cancer: Principles and Practice of Oncology, 2nd Edition. Updates 1987 (1):1-16

5 Simon JB: Occult blood screening for colorectal carcinoma: A critical review. Gastroenterology 1985 (88):820-837

6 Winawer SJ, Andrews M, Flehinger B et al: Progress report on controlled trial of fecal occult blood testing for the detection of colorectal neoplasia. Cancer 1980 (45):2959-2964

7 Gilbertsen VA, Church TR and Grewe FJ: The design of a study to assess occult-blood screening for colon cancer. J. Chron Dis 1980 (33):107-114

8 Flehinger BJ, Herbert E, Winawer SJ and Miller DG: Screening for colorectal cancer with fecal occult blood test and sigmoidoscopy: Preliminary report of the colon project of Sloan-Kettering Memorial Cancer Center and PMI-Strang Clinic. In: Chamberlain J and Miller AB (eds) Screening for Gastrointestinal Cancer. Hans Huber, Toronto 1988 pp 9-16

9 Gilbertsen VA, McHugh R, Schuman L and William SE: The early detection of colorectal cancers: a preliminary report of the results of the occult blood study. Cancer 1980 (45):2899-2901

10 Hardcastle JD, Thomas WM, Chamberlain J et al: Randomized controlled trial of fecal occult blood screening for colorectal cancer. The results of the first 107,349 subjects. Lancet 1989 (1):1160-1164

11 Kewenter J, Björk S, Haglind E et al: Screening and rescreening for colorectal cancer: a controlled trial of fecal occult blood testing in 27,700 subjects. Cancer 1988 (62):645-651

12 Kronborg C, Feuger O et al: Initial mass screening for colorectal cancer with fecal occult blood test. Scand J Gastroenterol 1987 (22):677-686

13 Hertz RE, Deddish MR and Day E: Value of periodic examinations in detecting cancer of the rectum and colon. Postgrad Med 1960 (27):290-294

14 Gilbertsen VA: Proctosigmoidoscopy and polypectomy in reducing the incidence of rectal cancer. Cancer 1974 (34):936-939

15 Selby JV, Friedman GD and Collen MF: Sigmoidoscopy and mortality from colorectal cancer: the Kaiser Permanent Multiphasic Evaluation Study. J Clin Epidemiol 1988 (41):427-434

16 Friedman GD, Collen MF and Fireman BH: Multiphasic health checkup evaluation: a 16-year follow-up. J Chron Dis 1986 (39):453-463

17 Leinicke JL, Dodds WJ, Hogan WJ et al: A comparison of colonoscopy and roentgenography for detecting polypoid lesions of the colon. Gastrointest Radiol 1977 (2):125-128

18 Hogan WJ, Stewart ET, Greenen JE et al: A prospective comparison of the accuracy of colonoscopy vs. air-barium contrast exam for detection of colonic polypoid lesions. Gastrointest Endosc 1977 (23):230-236

19 Ott DJ, Ablin AS, Gelfand DW et al: Predictive value of a diagnosis of colonic polyp on the double-contrast barium enema. Gastrointest Radiol 1983 (8):75-80

20 Anderson DF: Risk in families of patients with colon cancer. In: Winawer SJ, Schottenfeld D, Sherlock P (eds) Colorectal Cancer: Prevention, Epidemiology and Screening. Raven Press, New York 1980 pp 109-115

21 Duncan JL and Kyle J: Family incidence of carcinoma of the colon and rectum in North-East Scotland. Gut 1982 (23):169-171

22 Lovett E: Family studies in cancer of the colon and rectum. Br J Surg 1976 (63):13-18

23 Macklin M: Inheritance of cancer of the stomach and large intestine in man. JNCI 1960 (24):551-571

24 Woolf CM, Richards RC and Gardner EJ: Occasional discrete polyps of the colon and rectum showing an inherited tendency in a kindred. Cancer 1955 (8):403-408

25 Guillem JG, Neugut AI, Forde KA et al: Colonic neoplasms in asymptomatic first-degree relatives of colon cancer patients. Am J Gastroenterol 1988 (83):271-273

26 Burt RW, Bishop DT, Cannon LA et al: Dominant inheritance of adenomatous colonic polyps and colorectal cancer. N Engl J Med 1985 (312):1540-1544

27 Cannon LA, Skolnick MH, Bishop DT et al: Common inheritance of susceptibility to colonic adenomatous

polyps and associated colorectal cancers. N Engl J Med 1988 (319):533-537
28 Weber W, Vögtli B, Buser M et al: Vergleich der Tumorinzidenz bei 251 Verwandten ersten Grades von 50 Patienten mit kolorektalen Karzinomen mit derjenigen der Basler Bevölkerung. Schweiz Med Wschr 1985 (115):1005-1006
29 Murday V: Screening for colorectal cancer based on family history. In: Weber W, Laffer UT, Dürig M (eds) Hereditary Cancer and Preventive Surgery. Karger, Basel 1990 pp 34-38
30 Gryska PR and Cohen AM: Screening asymptomatic patients at high risk for colon cancer with full colonoscopy. Dis Colon Rectum 1987 (30):18-20
31 Guillem JG, Neugut AI, Forde KA et al: Colonic neoplasms in asymptomatic first-degree relatives of colon cancer patients. Am J Gastroenterol 1988 (83):271-273
32 Grossman S and Milos ML: Colonoscopic screening of persons with suspected risk factors for colon cancer. I. Family History. Gastroenterology 1988 (94):395-400
33 Orrom WJ, Brzezinski WS and Wiens EW: Heredity and colorectal cancer. A prospective, community-based, endoscopic study. Dis Colon Rectum 1990 (33):490-493
34 McConnell JC, Nizin JS and Slade MS: Colonoscopy in patients with a primary family history of colon cancer. Dis Colon Rectum 1990 (33):105-107
35 Ransohoff DF and Lang CA: Screening for colorectal cancer. N Engl J Med 1991 (325):37-41
36 Rex DK, Lehman GA, Hawes RH et al: Screening colonoscopy in asymptomatic average-risk persons with negative fecal occult blood tests. Gastroenterology 1991 (100):64-67

Preventive Surgery

Markus Zuber, Urban Laffer and Felix Harder

Department of Surgery, University of Basel, Switzerland

Preventive surgery is considered to be a secondary form of cancer prevention. This type of surgery is not primary prophylaxis because it does not eliminate the carcinogenic agent [1]. Prophylactic surgery prevents the formation of malignant tumours by removing tissue in patients who present in 2 different phases of potential development of a malignancy [2]. Firstly, patients with a positive familial history, gene carriers, with an increased risk, who are in a precancerous *condition* (the familial adenomatous polyposis (FAP) and the medullary thyroid carcinoma (MTC) of the multiple endocrine neoplasia syndrome (MEN-2a/2b) are the best known examples). Secondly, patients at a more advanced stage of disease, when a precancerous *lesion* has already established itself: for example, high-grade intraepithelial dysplasia, the so-called carcinoma *in situ* of the large bowel, breast, and other organs.
In the following sections attention will be paid to breast diseases, thyroid tumours associated with the MEN syndromes, and colon and rectum tumours in FAP.

Breast Diseases

In a list of precancerous conditions for breast cancer, all risk factors have to be included [3]. It has been shown that 35% of clinically healthy female members of breast cancer kindreds have proliferative breast disease defined by four-quadrant needle-aspiration cytology compared with 13% of controls. Genetic analysis suggests that genetic susceptibility causes both proliferative breast disease and breast cancer, the former being discussed as a risk factor itself [4].
With the growing use of screening programmes together with family history, frequent self-examination and mammography, detection of carcinoma *in situ* has increased considerably.
Ductal and lobular carcinoma *in situ* and Paget's disease of the nipple are precancerous lesions of the breast. It is well known that a non-invasive, intraductal or lobular carcinoma *in situ* may develop into either ductal or lobular invasive carcinoma.
A carcinoma *in situ* is a pre-invasive form of a high-grade neoplasia without light-microscopic evidence of invasion through the basement membrane into the neighbouring tissue.

Ductal Carcinoma* in Situ *(DCIS)

Thanks to the use of mammography for breast cancer screening, an increasing number of small, non-palpable tumours of less than 10 mm in diameter are being discovered [5,6]. Up to 59% of DCIS with clusters of microcalcifications are exclusively detected by mammography in the age group of around 50 years [7]. Four years after biopsy a 5% recurrence rate of invasive cancers (less than 25 mm) is found for DCIS [8]; after 3-10 years invasiveness is 28% [9]. The recurrence occurs in the ipsilateral breast and in most cases in the same quadrant where the primary lesion was removed.
The risk of invasive cancer depends on the multicentricity of the microcalcifications (32-78%). The risk increases when atypical ductal

proliferation, papillary or necrotic areas are found on histological examination. The comedo type seems to be the most aggressive [10,11]. Carpenter has postulated aneuploidy as a further risk factor [12].

In 48% of cases DCIS is diagnosed in the contralateral breast [13], but the cumulative risk of contralateral breast cancer has been reported to be only 12% 20 years after diagnosis of the primary carcinoma [14,15]. These observations suggest that not all DCIS progress to an invasive form of cancer. A caveat should be formulated regarding the interpretation of the above-mentioned, histologically revised diagnoses: these patients were treated for benign diseases with limited resections and with questionably clean margins.

The local recurrence rate for mammographically detected lesions treated with local excision is 8.5% after a short follow-up time of 43 months [16]. Fifty percent of these recurrences are invasive.

Axillary lymph-node metastases occur in 0-2% of DCIS. As the size of the lesions increases the chance of occult microinvasion through the basement membrane (detectable by electron-microscopic or immunohistochemical examination) and the risk of axillary lymph-node metastases augments.

Mastectomy has been the standard therapy for DCIS. The efficacy of this surgical procedure has been demonstrated in 3 studies (Table 1) [17-19]. Survival rates approach 100%.

However, DCIS can be treated successfully by breast conserving therapy (Table 2) [20-22,11,16]. Fisher's 2 figures represent a subgroup analysis of patients from the NSABP B06 study, who were later on microscopically re-classified as having only DCIS and not invasive carcinoma. Two cases treated with tumourectomy and radiotherapy showed recurrences as opposed to 5 cases treated with local excision alone.

In all trials except for Lagios' study [16], patients were admitted on the basis of palpable lesions and not of a cluster of microcalcifications detected by mammography.

Due to the small number of patients and the short follow-up, these results must be considered preliminary. A randomised multicentre trial (NSABP B17) is now under way to study the natural history of DCIS, the value of radiotherapy and the criteria for selecting patients for breast-conserving treatment.

Table 1. Radical treatment for ductal carcinoma in situ (DCIS)

		Mastectomy		
Author [ref]	N	Follow-up (yrs)	Local recurrence	Survival (%)
Ashikari [17]	74	11	0	100
Sunshine [18]	68	10	0	95
Farrow [19]	181	5-20	2	98

Table 2. Conservative treatment for ductal carcinoma in situ (DCIS)

		Tumourectomy with radiotherapy		
Author [ref]	N	Follow-up	Local recurrence	Survival (%)
Recht [20]	40	44 m	4	100
Zafrani [21]	54	55 m	3	98
Montague [22]	56	4 y	1	98
Fisher [11]	29	39 m	2 (7%)	100
		without radiotherapy		
Lagios [16]	71	43 m	6 (8.5%)	100
Fisher [11]	22	39 m	5 (23%)	100

Treatment Recommendations

Limited disease with a single cluster of microcalcifications on the mammogram, less than 25 mm in diameter (a figure which corresponds to Lagios' trial [16]) may be widely excised with histologically negative resection margins.

For lesions larger than 25 mm, tumourectomy and radiotherapy may be recommended, because the probability of occult microinvasion depends on tumour size. Clear resection margins are mandatory also in this breast-conserving treatment approach. For this treatment group Osteen proposed in 1988 axillary dissection, since in up to 2% regional lymph-node metastases were observed [23]. Close follow-up by mammography and physical examination is recommended. If on mammography a premalignant lesion occurs with multiple areas of suspicious microcalcification, it should be treated with mastectomy and axillary clearance.

Lobular Carcinoma in Situ *(LCIS)*

Screening mammography is usually of no help in discovering LCIS. It is the clinical appearance of a small palpable breast lump which leads to an excision biopsy. The patients are usually somewhat below the age of 50. In 80% the precancerous lesions are multicentric and in 47% bilateral [24]. Local recurrences occur in 22% as invasive carcinoma in the ipsilateral breast and in 15% in the contralateral breast [25]. Rosen's local recurrence rate is even higher with 33% invasive cancers after a follow-up period of 24 years, with an equal risk of both breasts and location anywhere in either breast [26].

Treatment Recommendations

These observations suggest the following therapeutic options for LCIS:

1. Bilateral mastectomy may be suitable for incurably anxious patients with a strong family history of breast cancer. This surgical approach is the only real prophylaxis.
2. Mastectomy of the affected side with blind contralateral biopsy has been advocated. Implicit in this approach is the belief that LCIS cells may become invasive and that blind biopsy will help identify those patients at risk of bilateral disease. Hard evidence that the risk for both breasts correlates with bilateral *in situ* disease is lacking. It is not clear whether LCIS is anything more than a marker for risk in both breasts [11].
3. Another option is local excision with clear margins without radiotherapy and without axillary clearance. A careful follow-up of both breasts with frequent clinical examination would seem preferable to bilateral mastectomy for most patients.

Paget's Disease of the Nipple

One to four percent of all breast diseases present with Paget's disease, namely with eczematoid changes in the nipple with itching, discharge, bleeding or combinations of the symptoms. Paget's disease is associated with a breast mass in 60%. Axillary lymph nodes are found to be negative when no breast lump is present [27]. If the mass is a non-invasive or invasive carcinoma, in 50% of the cases the axillary lymph nodes contain metastases. Osteen (1987) collected 46 cases in the literature and found only 3 recurrences after a short follow-up [28].

Treatment Recommendations

At present a breast-conserving procedure [28] with or without radiation is considered the therapy of choice for Paget's disease in the absence of a clinically or radiologically detected breast mass.
In case of an existing breast mass a modified radical mastectomy should be performed. In selected cases, depending on the localisation, size and histology of the lesion (examined by frozen section), tumourectomy (with total excision of the nipple complex) and radiotherapy is an alternative procedure.

Medullary Thyroid Carcinoma (MTC)

Medullary carcinoma arises in the parafollicular cells (C-cells). The tumour is familial in about 20% of cases and may be associated with the Multiple Endocrine Neoplasia Syndrome - Type 2. MTC comprises 5-12% of all thyroid cancers. MTC is not associated with the MEN-1 syndrome but with MEN-2a and 2b. MTC occurs always bilaterally. Pheochromocytoma is bilateral in 70% of cases [29]. Hyperparathyroidism with hyperplasia (seldom malignant disease) determines the difference between types 2a and 2b, except for a specific phenotype of 2b [30]. A newly diagnosed patient may be the index case of a new familial cluster and presents mostly with a carcinoma as a first sign of the disease. In familial cases, the lesions are generally bilateral [31]. Patients with

medullary carcinoma have a fair prognosis when the disease is limited to the thyroid gland. The prognosis is very poor when the malignancy is associated with lymph node metastases, which commonly occur in this type of cancer. The overall survival rate after 10 years of follow-up amounts to 50% [32].
An exciting development has been the use of provocation tests with calcium or pentagastrin for calcitonin as a tumour marker. This test can detect preclinical disease in patients at risk for familial medullary thyroid carcinoma. When, after stimulation, selective blood sampling from a inferior thyroid vein is performed and calcitonin levels are elevated, patients are found to have either C-cell hyperplasia or a minimal MTC that would otherwise have been undetectable [33]. This early disease is completely curable [34].
The use of linked DNA markers on chromosome 10 helps to identify gene carriers at risk for malignancy [31,35]. This finding may allow preventive thyroidectomy.

Treatment Recommendations

A precancerous lesion of C-cell hyperplasia and minimal medullary carcinoma diagnosed by means of elevated plasma calcitonin levels following stimulation is usually cured by thyroidectomy.
No longer considered as prophylactic surgery is the treatment of MTC by thyroidectomy and modified radical neck dissection.

Colorectal Disease

Various precancerous conditions with an increased risk for developing a malignancy exist in colorectal disease. The best example of such a condition is familial adenomatous polyposis [2].
Risk factors for colorectal cancer besides FAP are: Gardner, Turquot, Peutz-Jegher syndromes, Lynch syndrome type I and II, familial history of colorectal cancer, inflammatory bowel disease (ulcerative colitis), personal history of colorectal cancer, irradiation of the pelvis, precancerous lesions (e.g., carcinoma *in situ*) and, in general, age > 40 [36].

Familial Adenomatous Polyposis (FAP)

Ocular examination for congenital hypertrophy of the retinal pigment epithelium (CHRPE) is valuable for detecting carriers of the gene for FAP before symptoms develop [37]. Presymptomatic diagnosis can be comfirmed not only by linked DNA markers for identification of one FAP gene on chromosome 5, but also by identification of the adenomatous polyposis coli (APC) gene [38]. Members of kindreds with FAP can be tested pre- and postnatally for mutations of this gene [39].
For certain precancerous conditions and established lesions the question is not whether to operate or not, but only at what time and by which extension the surgical procedure should be carried out. The average age of onset of symptomatical FAP is about 20 years and the average age at which carcinoma is detected is 35. Cases have been recorded in which precancerous lesions were diagnosed at the age of 20. It would seem desirable to perform surgery between 16-20 years. In general this would mean to operate on phenotypically healthy patients [40].

Treatment Recommendations

The ideal treatment for FAP from the surgical oncology point of view would be a total proctocolectomy. The drawback of this surgical procedure is the establishment of a permanent ileostomy and consequent bladder and sexual malfunction.
A less drastic surgical procedure is colectomy with an ileorectal anastomosis. The polyps in the rectal stump are destroyed pre-, peri- or postoperatively. The risk of rectal cancer after abdominal colectomy for polyposis varies in a range of 7.5-59% of the cases. Moertel reported this high cancer rate 23 years after primary surgery [41]. Careful clinical follow-up with frequent endoscopy is essential for patients treated with less radical surgical procedures and thus still at risk for cancer.
The third operation, described by Parks and Nicholls in 1978 [42], consists of a colectomy with submucosal proctectomy in the rectal stump, followed by the construction of an ileal pouch which is pulled into the prepared rectal stump, so that an ileo-anal anastomosis can

be performed. Normal continence is achieved in over 90%. The risk of bladder and sexual dysfunction is low. More frequent evacuations (3-4 day and night) and pouch inflammation (in up to 30%) are disadvantages.

Concluding Remarks

Preventive surgery is an option in the case of increased risk conditions and precancerous lesions. Absolute indications for surgery of precancerous conditions are symptomless gene carriers of familial adenomatous polyposis and members of MEN-2a or 2b families with elevated plasma calcitonin levels after stimulation. In addition, all individuals at increased risk compared to the general population should remain under close and careful clinical observation in order not to miss the ideal point in time for preventive surgery. Exciting advances in the near future in fields such as molecular biology, cytogenetics, cellular immunology and protein chemistry will help identify these individuals at higher risk, so that accurate surgery can be performed at the optimal time point.

REFERENCES

1 Harder F: Prophylactic surgery. In: Weber W, Laffer UT, Dürig M (eds) Hereditary Cancer and Preventive Surgery. Basel, Karger 1990 pp 67-69

2 Gall FP, Hermanek P: Präventive Operationsindikationen bei Präcancerosen im Gastrointestinaltrakt. Chirurg 1987 (58): 228-233

3 Henderson IC, Harris JR, Kinne DW, Hellmann S: Cancer of the breast. In: DeVita VT, Hellmann S, Rosenberg SA (eds) Cancer. Principles and Practice of Oncology. Philadelphia, Lippincott 1989 3rd ed pp 1197-1268

4 Skolnik MH, Cannon-Albright LA, Goldgar DE et al: Inheritance of proliferative breast disease in breast cancer kindreds. Science (1990) 250: 1715-1720.

5 Schnitt SJ, Silen W, Sandowsky NL et al: Ductal carcinoma in situ (intraductal carcinoma) of the breast. N Engl J Med 1988 (318): 898-903

6 Cooke TG: Ductal carcinoma in situ: a new clinical problem. Br J Surg 1989 (76): 660-662

7 Baker LH: Breast cancer detection demonstration project: five year summary report. Cancer 1982 (32): 194-225

8 Lagios MD, Margolin FR, Westdahl PR, Rose MR: Mammographically detected duct carcinoma in situ. Cancer 1989 (63): 618-624

9 Page DL, Dupont WD, Rogers LW, Landenberger M: Intraductal carcinoma of the breast: follow up after biopsy only. Cancer 1982 (49): 751-758

10 Meyer JS. Cell kinetics of histologic variants of in situ breast carcinoma. Breast Cancer Res Treat 1986 (7): 171-180

11 Fisher ER, Sass R, Fisher B et al: Pathologic findings from the National Surgical Adjuvant Breast Project (Project 6) I. Intraductal Carcinoma (DCIS). Cancer 1986 (57): 197-208

12 Carpenter R, Gibbs N, Matthew J, Cooke T: Importance of cellular DNA content in premalignant breast disease and preinvasive carcinoma of the female breast. Br J Surg 1987 (74): 905-906

13 Albert CE, Wellings S: The prevalence of carcinoma in situ in normal and cancer associated breasts. Hum Pathol 1985 (16): 796-807

14 Robbins GF, Berg JW: Bilateral primary breast cancers: a prospective clinicopathological study. Cancer 1964 (17): 1501-1527.

15 Fisher ER, Gregorio R, Fisher B: The pathology of invasive breast cancer: a syllabus derived from the findings of the National Surgical Adjuvant Breast Protocol (Protocol 4). Cancer 1975 (36): 1-85

16 Lagios MD: Human breast precancers: current status. Cancer Surv 1983 (2): 383- 402

17 Ashikari R, Huvos AG, Snyder RE: Prospective study of non-infiltrating carcinoma of the breast. Cancer 1977 (39): 435-439

18 Sunshine JA, Moseley HS, Fletcher WS, Krippaehne WW: Breast carcinoma in situ: a retrospective review of 112 cases with a minimum 10 year follow up. Am J Surg 1985 (150): 44-51

19 Farrow JH: Current concepts in the detection and the treatment of the earliest of the early breast cancers. Cancer 1970 (25): 468-477

20 Recht A, Danoff BS, Solin LJ: Intraductal carcinoma of the breast: results of treatment with excisional biopsy and irradiation. J Clin Oncol 1985 (3): 1339-1343

21 Zafrani B, Fourquet A, Viloq JR, Legal M, Calle R: Conservative management of intraductal breast carcinoma with tumorectomy and radiation therapy. Cancer 1986 (57): 1299-1301

22 Montague ED: Conservation surgery and radiation therapy in the treatment of operable breast cancer. Cancer 1984 (53 Suppl 3): 700-704

23 Osteen RT: Surgery for non-invasive breast cancer. In: Cohn LH (ed) Controversies in Surgery. Syllabus, Harvard Medical School, Continuing Education, Department of Surgery, Brigham and Women's Hospital, Boston, 1988

24 Olbrisch RR: Praeventive Operationsindikationen in der Mammachirurgie. Chirurg 1987 (58): 234-238

25 Haagensen CD, Lane N, Lattes R, Bodian C: Lobular neoplasia (so-called lobular carcinoma in situ) of the breast. Cancer 1978 (42): 737-769

26 Rosen PP, Liebermann PH,Braun DW, Kosloff C, Adair F: Lobular carcinoma in situ of the breast: detailed analysis of 99 patients with average follow up of 24 years. Am J Surg Pathol 1978 (2): 225-251

27 Nance FC, DeLoach, Welsh RA: Paget's disease of the breast. Ann Surg 1970 (171): 864-874

28 Osteen RT. Paget's disease of the nipple. In: Harris JR, Hellman S, Henderson IC, Linne DW (eds)

Breast Diseases. Philadelphia, Lippincott 1987 pp 589-595
29 Carney JA, Sizemore GW, Sheps SG: Adrenal medullary disease in multiple endocrine neoplasia type 2. Am J Clin Pathol 1976 (66): 279
30 Keiser HR, Beaven MA, Doppmann J et al: Sipple's syndrome: medullary thyroid carcinoma, pheochromocytoma and parathyroid disease. Ann Intern Med 1973 (78): 561
31 Lips CJM, Struyvenberg A, van der Slys Veer J, van Vroonhoven: Hereditary malignant disease of the endocrine system. In: Weber W, Laffer UT, Dürig M (eds) Hereditary Cancer and Preventive Surgery. Basel, Karger 1990 pp 77-83
32 Norton JA, Doppmann JL, Jensen RT: Cancer of the endocrine system. In: DeVIta VT, Hellman S, Rosenberg SA (eds) Cancer. Principles and Practice of Oncology. Philadelphia, Lippincott 1989 3rd ed pp 1269-1344
33 Wells SA, Baylin SB, Johnsrude JS et al: Thyroid venous catheterisation in the early diagnosis of familial medullary thyroid carcinoma. Ann Surg 1982 (196): 505
34 Wells SA, Baylin SB, Leight GS et al: The importance of the early diagnosis in patients with hereditary medullary thyroid carcinoma. Ann Surg 1982 (195): 505
35 Sobol H, Narod SA, Nakamura Y, Lenoir GM et al: Screening for MEN type 2a with DNA-polymorphism analysis. N Engl J Med 1989 (321): 996-1001
36 Cohen AM, Shank B, Friedman MA: Colorectal cancer. In: DeVita VT, Hellmann S, Rosenberg SA. Cancer. Principles and Practice of Oncology. Philadelphia, Lippincott 1989 3rd ed pp 895-964
37 Chapman PD, Church W, Burn J, Gunn A: Congenital hypertrophy of retinal pigment epthelium: a sign of familial adenomatous polyposis. Br Med J 1989 (298): 353-354
38 Groden J, Thliveris A, Samowitz W et al: Identification and characterisation of the familial adenomatous polyposis coli gene. Cell 1991 (66): 589-600
39 Kinzler KW, Nilbert MC, Su LK et al: Identification of FAP locus genes from chromosome 5q21. Science 1991 (253): 661-665
40 Goligher J: Familial polyposis. In: Goligher J (ed). Surgery of the Anus, Rectum and the Colon. London, Balliere Tindall 1984 5th ed pp 399-425
41 Moertel CG, Hill JR, Adson MA: Management of multiple polyposis of the large bowel. Cancer 1971 (28): 160
42 Parks AG, Nicholls RJ: Restorative proctocolectomy without ileostomy for ulcerative colitis. Br Med J 1978 (2): 85-88

Desmoids in Gardner's Syndrome: A Challenge for Surgeons

S. Martinoli, L. Mariani and A. Goldhirsch

Department of Surgery and Division of Oncology, Ospedale Civico, Lugano, Switzerland

Gardner's first description [1] of the association of familial adenomatous polyposis (FAP) with osteomas and skin lesions (1951-1953) was followed by steadily increasing discoveries of other extracolonic manifestations, such as upper gastrointestinal lesions (fundic gland polyps, true gastric and duodenal adenomas) [2], desmoid tumours, retinal changes and other more unusual associations like brain tumours [3], papillary carcinoma in the thyroid [4] and hepatoblastomas [5].

In a series reported by Bussey [6] from the Polyposis Register of St. Mark's Hospital, upper gastrointestinal malignancy has become the most common FAP-related cause of death. According to the same paper, desmoid tumours seem to become an important cause of morbidity and mortality.

Desmoids are a not infrequent cause of anuria or of a definitive anenteric condition. They can jeopardise vital structures like intestinal vasculature or impair the function of major nerval structures. The following 4 cases illustrate abundantly their somewhat deleterious pathology.

Case 1

A 41-year-old man with neither previous disease nor family history comes to the emergency ward with a bowel obstruction. After a short conservative treatment, laparotomy is performed. At operation (Fig. 1), the radix mesenterii is found to be infiltrated by a large and badly delimited mass, encircling the vessels of the whole small bowel. A resection of the whole mass (2.5 kg in weight) is done. An end-to-end anastomosis between distal duodenum and transverse colon has to be performed. After an uneventful postoperative recovery, the patient is given an indwelling nu-

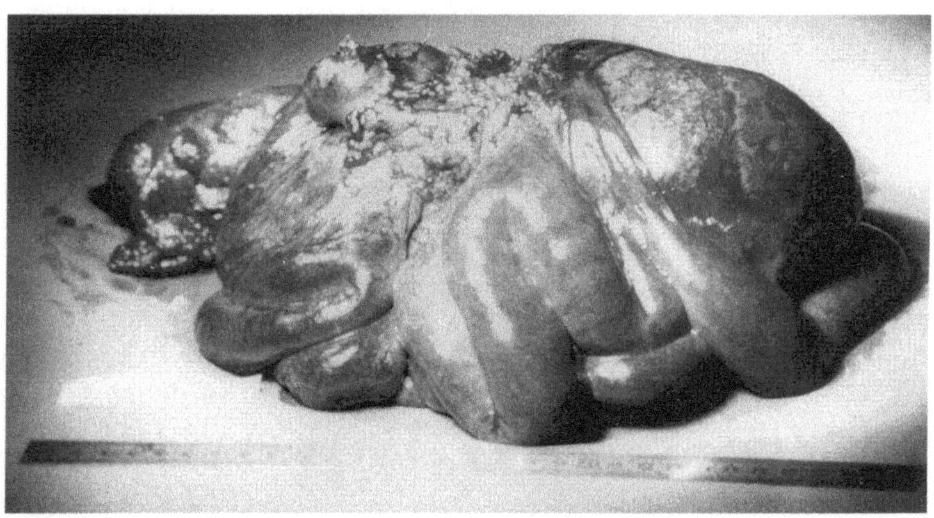

Fig. 1. The resected specimen, 2.5 kg in weight, showing invasion of the mesentery and total fusion with the whole small bowel

tritional reservoir. Colonoscopy shows that the residual colon is free of polyps but at gastroscopy the whole stomach is found to be lined by a jungle of small polyps. A strict limitation of sugar and fat in the parenteral nutrition leads to the disappearance of a temporary jaundice. The patient is now alive and in good health 2.5 years after the desmoid resection. He is able to eat and resorb more and more oral nutrition.

Case 2

A 35-year-old woman belonging to a known Gardner family underwent subtotal colectomy with ileorectal anastomosis because she was found to have more than three 1-cm polyps. One year later a mass is clinically suspected. The left ureter and kidney calyx become more and more dilated (Fig. 2) due to the mass compressing the ureter before entering the bladder. After a short course of toremifen without any relief of the urinary obstruction, laparotomy is performed. A mass measuring 10 cm is found invading the superior mesenteric axis; the mass is totally inexcisable without sacrificing the whole small bowel. A second mass is found in the left lower retroperitoneal space, encircling and firmly compressing the left ureter. A stent can just be passed into the bladder and the kidney calyx. Six months later the two desmoids are stable, even in light regression with concomitant medroxyprogesterone and toremifen therapy. Kidney function is symmetrical and good. The stent has to be changed every two months.

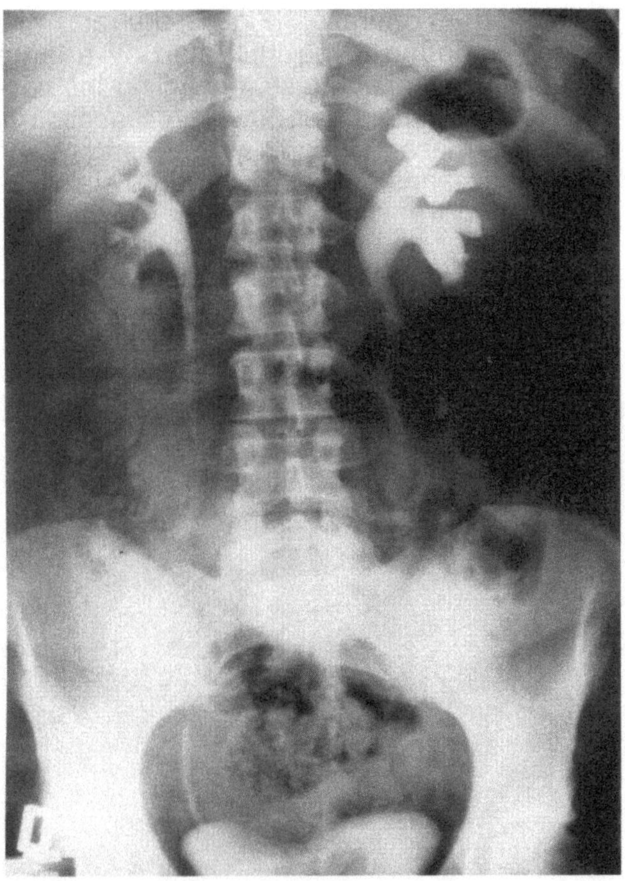

Fig. 2. The desmoid is compressing the left distal ureter, causing hydronephrosis of the left kidney calyx

Case 3

A 55-year-old woman lost her father and four of her aunts due to intestinal cancer. One of her sisters had a desmoid after colectomy and died. Following rectal bleeding and colonoscopy, colectomy with ileorectal anastomosis is performed. More than 100 partially dysplastic polyps are found. Two years later, during follow-up, a mass is discovered in the abdomen. A short period of observation follows, in the hope that the recent cessation of menses would check the progression.

One year later, the mass is seen to enlarge more and more and a CT-scan (Fig. 3) confirms its grotesque expansion. In a desperate attempt to palliate the ongoing bowel obstruction, laparotomy is performed. The mass is infiltrating the whole radix mesenterii and is totally inoperable. The patient dies 6 months later after ineffective treatment with a somatostatin-analogue and an attempt with tamoxifen.

Case 4

A 35-year-old man had a clavicle fracture in 1977. In 1983 he consults his doctor because a dense tissue scar can be palpated below the right clavicle. The pathologist describes the biopsy as "reparative tissue, non-suspect for aggressive behaviour". Subsequently, the patient develops slowly progressive symptoms of brachial plexus compression. A CT-scan made in 1988 (Fig. 4) shows a definitely

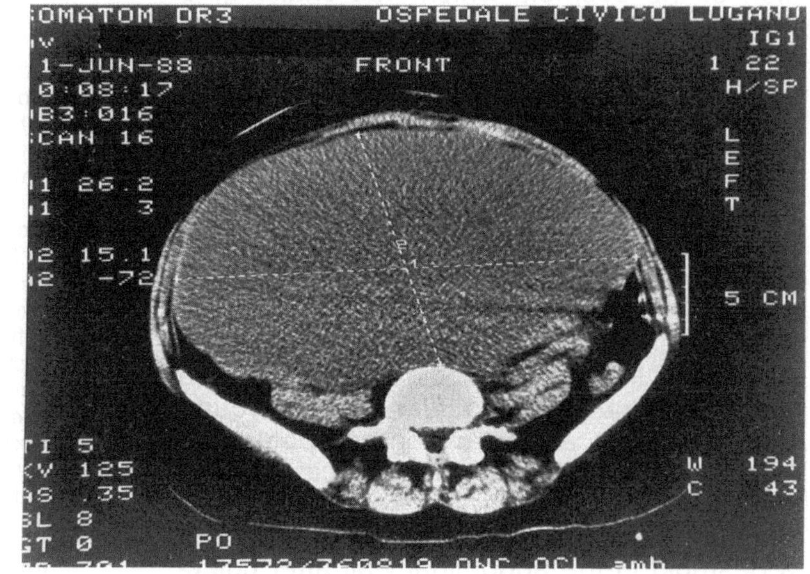

Fig. 3. CT scan of the giant desmoid of the mesentery

expanding infraclavian mass between the first two ribs and the pectoralis muscle. Radical resection of the tumour with thoracic wall, M. pectoralis and clavicle, is performed. At operation the brachial plexus is still not encircled or touched by the tumour, even though the subclavian vein has to be resected for radicality. Some doubt exists about radicality because of the proximity of the tumour to the fibrous sheath of the brachial plexus. High-voltage radiotherapy to 54 Gy is well tolerated. The patient is now alive and well with a well functioning right arm. He has been recognised to be a member of a numerous family showing Gardner's syndrome. Colonoscopy could not reveal polyps so far but his stomach is full of gastric fundic gland polyps.

Discussion

In Case 1 the desmoid was the first manifestation of the syndrome. In Case 2 the operation seemed to have triggered the progres-

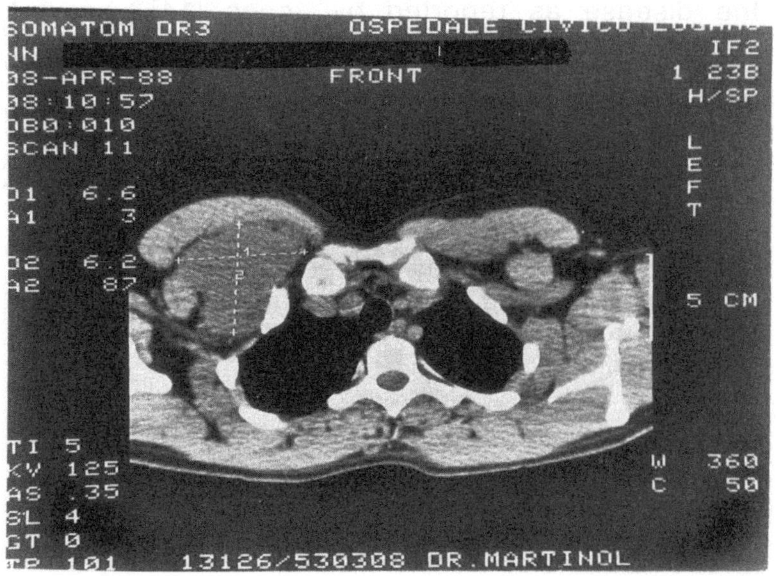

Fig. 4. In CT scan the expanding feature of the infraclavear desmoid can be clearly observed

sion of the desmoid which was challenging the renal function of the patient. In both cases, surgery was only able to palliate the unusual aggressiveness of the desmoid. In Case 3 a striking remark must be made: without prophylactic colectomy our patient would probably have survived longer. The mother of our Case 2 lived to 65 with polyps but without malignant degeneration. Prophylactic surgery prevents early death from colorectal cancer but possibly enhances extracolonic mortality by triggering the explosion of life-threatening desmoids. In Case 4 it took 7 years until the physician was able to identify the young man's mass as an expanding and potentially hazardous tumour. The histological appearance was misleading. This young man was the son of a woman with FAP who developed a desmoid in the abdominal wall after colectomy and the brother of the lady of Case 2. It was mandatory in this case to avoid recurrence in the wound scar. Radiotherapy was successful in consolidating surgical excision. Desmoids do not metastasise but may infiltrate surrounding tissues. The recurrence rate is about 25-65% [6]. Some infrequent spontaneous regression is reported [7,8]. Very spectacular regressions have been observed with administration of sulindac, progesterone, indomethacin, ascorbate, prednison, tamoxifen and toremifen [9-11]. The frequency of desmoids in FAP individuals varies between 4% and 13% [12,13]. Surgery has to be considered as the first choice of treatment in the case of resectability or obstruction. However, surgery is not infrequently unable to eradicate the disease as reported by Jones [14]. Whichever procedure is chosen for the prophylaxis of impending colonic cancer, it is very important to remember that the FAP patient still requires lifelong follow-up because of the possibility of developing extracolonic and sometimes life-threatening manifestations. The expected oncological benefit from colon surgery should be weighed against the possible triggering effect of surgery on desmoid formation in particulary desmoid-prone families.

REFERENCES

1 Gardner EJ and Richards RC: Multiple cutaneous and subcutaneous lesions occurring simultaneously with hereditary intestinal polyposis and esteomas. Am J Hum Genet 1953 (5):139-147

2 Watanabe H, Enjoji M, Yao T and Oshato K: Gastric lesions in familial adenomatosis coli: their incidence and histological analysis. Human Pathology 1978 (9):269-283

3 Turcot J, Despres JP and St. Pierre F: Malignant tumors of the central nervous system associated with familial polyposis of the colon. Dis Colon Rectum 1959 (2):465

4 Plail RO, Glazer G, Thomson JPS and Bussey HJR: Adenomatous polyposis: an association with carcinoma of the thyroid? Br J Surg 1985 (72):1385

5 Garber GE, Li FP and Kingston JE: Hepatoblastoma and familial adenomatous polyposis. JNCI 1988 (80):1626-1628

6 Bussey HJR, Evers AA, Ritchie SM and Thompson JPS: The rectum in adenomatous polyposis: the St. Mark's policy. Br J Surg 1985 (72):529-531

7 Reitamo JJ, Scheinin TM and Häyry P: The desmoid syndrome: new aspects in the cause, pathogenesis and treatment of the desmoid tumor. Am J Surg 1986 (151):230-237

8 Stevenson JK: Unfamiliar aspects of familial polyposis coli. Am J Surg 1986 (152):81-86

9 Eagel BA, Zentler-Munro and Smith JE: Mesenteric desmoid tumors in Gardner's syndrome - Review of medical treatments. Postgrad Med J 1989 (65):497-501

10 Waddell WR: Treatment of intraabdominal and abdominal wall desmoid tumors with drugs that affect the metabolism of cyclic 3'5'adenosin monophosphate. Ann Surg 1975 (81):299

11 Wilson AJ, Baum M, Singh L and Kangas L: Antioestrogen therapy of pure mesenchymal tumour. Lancet 1987 (i):508

12 Bussey HJR: Familial Polyposis Coli: Family Studies, Histopathology, Differential Diagnosis and Results of Treatment. Baltimore: Johns Hopkins University Press 1975

13 Lotfi AM, Dozois RR, Gordon H et al: Mesenteric fibromatosis complicating familial adenomatous polyposis: predisposing factors and result of treatment. Int J Colorect Dis 1989 (4):30-36

14 Jones IT, Fazio VW and Weakly FL: Desmoid tumors in familial polyposis coli. Ann Surg 1986 (204):94-97

Radiation and Cancer Prevention

J.M. Haefliger

Oncology - Radiotherapy Department, Communal Hospital, La Chaux-de-Fonds, Switzerland

Radiotherapy is a treatment that consists in destroying, by means of ionising radiation, an objectively visible and measurable tumour. Therefore, the answer to the question, "Does radiotherapy play a role in cancer prevention?" must definitely be: "No". On the contrary, ionising radiation is one of the most important agents involved in carcinogenesis. Furthermore, radiation is also known to be mutagenic. Even at therapeutic doses, it may induce severe side effects in normal tissues. Consequently, we may conclude that, in terms of prevention, exposure to ionising radiation should be avoided.

However, it may be useful to mention here that some recent reports have raised the surprising possibility that very low doses of ionising radiation may not be harmful and could even have certain benefits, a phenomenon known as hormesis [1,2]. Such new observations tend to show that DNA repair or immune cell production may be enhanced by very low doses of radiation. Nevertheless, this is, as yet, just a hypothesis and the commonly accepted health policy which stresses the importance of avoiding any exposure to radiation is still fully valid.

Carcinogenic Role of Radiation

Ionising radiation is probably the most thoroughly studied human carcinogen. Numerous epidemiological studies conducted on different populations that were accidentally or therapeutically exposed to low or high doses of ionising radiation have been published [3-5]. Research has been done on animals and cell cultures to reach a better understanding of the complicated and not yet fully understood mechanisms that lead to malignant transformation. All conclude that it is important to avoid any unnecessary exposure to ionising radiation. As a therapeutic agent it is primarily used for the treatment of patients with proven malignant tumours; the ultimate aim of radiation therapy is to permanently inhibit the proliferation of cancer cells.

This very restrictive approach is explained by several observations:

a) Any dose of radiation can induce cancer.

The literature shows that there is no threshold dose below which no risk of radiation-induced cancer can be accepted [5]. Any exposure to radiation, even at very low doses, may be sufficient to increase the risk of developing cancer years later. According to Jablon [6], exposure to ionising radiation is responsible for as many as 3% of the annual cancer incidence in the U.S.A.

b) Ionising radiation does not induce characteristic types of cancer.

Radiation-induced cancers cannot be distinguished from non radiation-induced ones. Only precise epidemiological studies on cancer incidence in exposed and non-exposed populations may provide some answers. However, definite conclusions will be difficult to draw without an evaluation of the role of simultaneous exposure to other carcinogenic agents such as tobacco, alcohol, nutritional habits or industrial pollutants.

c) The latency between exposure to radiation and diagnosis of cancer is variable. The minimal latency period between exposure to radiation and diagnosis of cancer is generally 8 to 10 years, sometimes even longer, up to 30 years. In specific situations, particularly for radiogenic breast and lung cancer, it seems that age-dependent factors may influence the radiation-induced expression of the disease. The cancer incidence is increased in exposed versus non-exposed populations.

d) The incidence of any type of cancer may be increased after exposure to radiation.

Several studies conclude that the incidence of nearly all types of cancer may be increased after exposure to ionising radiation. Breast, thyroid and bone marrow, however, appear to be the most radio-sensitive tissues. As age at exposure may be the most important host factor affecting subsequent cancer risk, it seems important to prevent any unnecessary exposure of patients - expecially young patients - to ionising radiation. There should be no useless radiological examinations and no therapeutic irradiation for inflammatory or benign conditions if these can be diagnosed or treated otherwise. Glynn [7] points out that teenage girls exposed to X-rays are likely to have a greater lifelong breast cancer risk than older women exposed to the same doses. Thus, shielding during dental and medical examinations, particularly in the age of breast development, is very important.

c) The risks per cGy are not the same for all organs [3].

The risks depend on several factors, such as physical characteristics of the radiation, the rate at which energy is deposited in tissues, the type of fractionation of the dose, the age of the patient, the organ in question, the endocrinological status. According to Boice, with respect to breast cancer neither fractionation nor radiation quality seem to affect either the shape of the dose-effect curves or the estimated radiation risk. Here, induction of cancer seems mainly hormonally mediated and ionising radiation could act as a cofactor of carcinogenesis.

At present, in spite of the numerous studies carried out, we still do not have any clear evidence of a relationship between the natural incidence of a given malignancy and the radiosensitivity of specific tissues or organs. For example, the natural incidence of colorectal cancer is high but its relative risk per cGy is low; the opposite is true for thyroid cancer, which has a low natural incidence but a high relative risk per cGy.

Radiation-Induced Damage in Normal Tissues

The damage induced by low doses of radiation is mainly carcinogenic and mutagenic. At therapeutic doses, numerous adverse effects in normal tissues can be noticed. They may appear early following exposure, may be repaired in some situations, but may also be permanent and compromise the quality of life of the patient.

Each organ possesses its proper tolerance to radiation: tolerance is low for organs such as testis, bone marrow, kidney and liver, whereas it is higher for the gut and soft tissues. Radio-induced lesions in these tissues may be responsible for more severe complications when subsequent infections or accidental or surgical trauma occur. The reason for this is that after therapeutic irradiation the tissues involved always sustain subclinical residual injury [9]. Furthermore, unnecessary irradiation may make further irradiation treatment impossible even though this may be indicated.

We will not present here a review of radiation-induced pathologies but just mention some common situations such as atrophy of the skin, damage to the epithelia of the gastrointestinal tract disturbing their physiological functions, kidney damage causing hypertension, lung damage with anticipated functional loss, disturbances in immune responses. There is an extensive review on these conditions by Awwad [9].

Use of Irradiation in Non-Cancerous Situations

Therapeutic application of ionising radiation primarily concerns the treatment of proven malignancies. The use of radiation for benign diseases, once common, is now rarely indicated except for a few radiosensitive benign diseases or for life-threatening radiosensitive conditions that cannot be treated in any other way such as pterygium of the eye, exophthalmos in patients with Graves' disease, orbital pseudotumours, keloids, cavernous haemangioma of the liver, vertebral haemangioma, bursitis, tendonitis, desmoids, fibromatosis, Peyronie's disease, nasopharyngeal angiofibroma, ectopic bone formation, etc. None of these diseases is precancerous. If radiation has to be applied for these conditions, the rules of the Committee on Radiation Treatment of Benign Disease of the Bureau of the Radiological Health have to be respected [10].

1. Before institution of therapy, account should be taken of the quality of radiation, total dose, overall time, underlying organs at risk, shielding factors.
2. Infants and children should be treated with ionising radiation only in very exceptional cases and after careful evaluation of the potential risk compared with the expected benefit.
3. Direct irradiation of the skin areas overlying organs that are prone to late effects (thyroid, gonads, bone marrow, breast) should be avoided.
4. Meticulous radiation protection techniques should be used in all instances.
5. The depth of penetration of the X-ray beam should be chosen in accordance with the depth of the pathologic process.

These rules almost totally exclude the use of ionising radiation to treat precancerous lesions or to prevent high-risk individuals from developing cancer. However, in a few situations the therapeutic use of radiation has been discussed:

a) Lentigo maligna or melanotic precancerosis [1], if surgery is contraindicated, because, unlike other types of melanoma, this disease is extremely radiosensitive.

b) Ovarian irradiation to induce prophylactic castration in premenopausal women with breast carcinoma. This is a controversial topic, although Nissen-Meyer advocates its use [12]. We would not recommend it today since it is known that there is a 3-fold risk of developing ovarian cancer 30 years after this therapy.

c) Intraductal breast carcinoma is a particular disease in which postoperative radiation may cause a significant reduction in local recurrence. It is perhaps the best example of a disease in which preventive radiation is possible, if we accept Haagensen's theory that intraductal breast carcinoma is a precancerous condition. This theory, however, is not unequivocal.

Conclusions

Our review shows that radiation cannot be considered as a therapeutic agent in cancer prevention. Since ionising radiation increases the risk of radio-induced cancer, any exposure should be avoided if no precise indication can be given, especially in populations at particular risk of developing cancer. This recommendation is the unique contribution of the radio-oncologist whose primary concern is the treatment of proven malignancies.

REFERENCES

1 Sagan LA: On radiation, paradigms and hormesis. Science 1989 (245):574

2 Wolf S: Are radiation-induced effects hormetic. Science 1989 (245):575

3 Boice JD: Cancer following medical irradiation. Cancer 1981 (47):1081-1090

4 Weber W (ed): Ionisierende Strahlen und Krebs. Ligue Suisse contre le Cancer. Berne 1990

5 Health Effects of Exposure to Low Levels of Ionizing Radiation. BEIR V. National Academy Press, Washington 1990

6 Jablon S, Bailar JC: The contribution of ionizing radiation to cancer mortality in the United States. Prev Med 1980 (9):227-230

7 Glynn TJ, Manley MW, Cullen JW, Mayer WJ: Cancer prevention through physician intervention. Sem Oncol 1990 (17):391-401

8 Boice JD Jr, Land CE, Shore RE et al: Risk of breast cancer following low dose radiation exposure. Radiology 1979 (131):589-597

9 Awwad HK: Radiation Oncology. Radiobiological and Physiological Perspectives. The boundary zone between clinical radiotherapy and fundamental radiobiology and physiology. Kluwer Academic Publishers, Boston, Dordrecht, London 1990

10 Bureau of Radiological Health: A review of the use of ionizing radiation for the treatment of benign disease, Vol. I. US Department of Health, Education and Welfare, Rockville MD 1977 pp 1-2

11 Schnyder UW, Sigg C: Management of hereditary melanoma and precursors. In: Weber W, Laffer UT, Durig M (eds) Hereditary Cancer and Preventive Surgery. Karger, Basel 1990 pp 84-92

12 Nissen-Meyer R: Primary breast cancer: The effect of primary ovarian irradiation. Ann Oncol 1991 (2):343-346

Chemoprevention

W. Weber and S. Kubba

Clinical Cancer Aetiology Unit, Basel, Switzerland

With the aging of the population cancer mortality is increasing. Cancer treatment is making progress - steadily but slowly. Therefore, the therapy for late disease needs to be complemented by other approaches. In recent years, the possibility has been raised that pharmacologic agents or nutritional modification can prevent the development of human neoplasia, slow down its progression, or make it regress. Basic research has corroborated this concept [1], and clinical trials have shown that chemopreventive agents can be effective in controlling oral leukoplakia, [2,3], solar keratosis [4], skin cancer [5] and second primary head and neck squamous cell carcinomas [6]. High fibre intake leads to a decrease in the number of polyps in patients with familial adenomatous polyposis [7]. The initial choice of chemopreventive agents for clinical trials has been limited to a few compounds and has been dictated by epidemiologic and laboratory data available in the late 1970s and by the rigid requirement of the use of a "safe" compound in normal or nearly normal populations [8]. The safety level required should be related to the level of risk [9]. For example, if the study population is composed of normal or nearly normal subjects (such as volunteers with a history of one polyp), very few or no side effects will be tolerated by either subjects or staff. In contrast, if the subjects are at high risk (e.g., have a history of familial polyposis, or second tumours), considerable side effects may be acceptable.
Another major consideration in the development of chemopreventive agents is the assessment of efficacy. Unless at least a few side effects are manifest, one might argue that there is no biologic activity. The determination of levels of the compound in serum or relevant tissues or the modulation of relevant biomarkers will therefore be important [10].
Only beta carotene, the retinoids, folic acid, and vitamins C and E have been used so far in phase III clinical chemoprevention trials. The retinoids are the longest-studied and currently most promising chemopreventive agents for epithelial cancers [15]. The development of new classes of compounds with minimal toxicity, targeted pharmacologic distribution, and the ability to modulate relevant biomarkers used as intermediate end points will be a major achievement that may lead to even more effective compounds.
On the basis of promising preclinical anticarcinogenic activity, hundreds of potential chemopreventive compounds have been identified from dietary sources (such as vegetables and garlic). A formal decision-making network has been organised by the U.S. National Cancer Institute to deal with the large numbers of compounds that will be discovered by screening [8]. There are at present about 12 large phase III or IV cancer-control clinical chemoprevention trials being conducted in the United States and another 5 elsewhere. These studies involve subjects at high risk for cancers of the skin, colorectum, cervix, breast, lung, and other organs, who are being treated with retinol, beta carotene, isotretinoin, 4-hydroxy-phenylretinamide and other compounds [8]. These trials involve more than 100,000 subjects. If even a few provide positive results, the manner in which we view the management of cancer is likely to undergo a fundamental change. The next few years will see the maturation of many of these clinical chemoprevention trials. Results are eagerly anticipated.

Taking a family history is the simplest method to identify healthy persons at high cancer risk [11,12]. In breast cancer it is the most easily obtainable risk marker for multicentre prevention studies. Women with a first-degree relative developing breast cancer before age 50 or 2 first-degree relatives after age 50 have a 3 to 4-fold increase in life-time breast cancer risk [13]. In these women a carefully conducted randomised pilot study with tamoxifen is ongoing at the Royal Marsden Hospital in London. This has shown that tamoxifen is well tolerated with a compliance of around 80% for both placebo and treated groups at 2 years [14].
Furthermore, biochemical monitoring of lipids and clotting factors indicate that tamoxifen may reduce the risk of cardiovascular deaths. A phase III tamoxifen prevention study is now planned in high-risk women identified by family history. Switzerland will be able to participate thanks to financial support from the Swiss Cancer League.

REFERENCES

1 Bertram JS, Kolonel LN, Meyskens FL Jr: Rationale and strategies for chemoprevention of cancer in humans. Cancer Res 1987 (47):3012-3031

2 Hong WK, Endicott J, Itri LM et al: 13-cis-Retinoic acid in the treatment of oral leukoplakia. N Engl J Med 1986 (315):1501-1505

3 Garewal HS, Meyskens FL Jr, Killen D et al: Response of oral leukoplakia to beta carotene. J Clin Oncol 1990 (8):1715-1720

4 Moriarty M, Dunn J, Darragh A et al: Etretinate in the treatment of actinic keratosis. Lancet 1982 (1):364-365

5 Moshell AN: Preventionof skin cancer in xeroderma pigmentosum with oral isotretinoin. Cutis 1989 (43):485-490

6 Hong WK, Lippman SM, Loretta MI et al: Prevention of second primary tumours with isotretinoin in squamous-cell carcinoma of the head and neck. N Engl J Med 1990 (323):795-801

7 De Cosse JJ, Miller HH, Lesser ML: Effect of wheat fiber and vitamins C and E on rectal polyps in patients with familial adenomatous polyposis. JNCI 1989 (81):1290-1297

8 Boone CW, Kelloff GJ, Malone WE: Identification of candidate cancer chemoprevention agents and their evaluation in animal models and human clinical trials: a review. Cancer Res 1990 (50):2-9

9 Meyskens FL, Jr: Coming of age - the chemoprevention of cancer. N Engl J Med 1990 (323):825-827

10 Lippman SM, Lee JS, Lotan R, Hittelman W, Wargowich MJ, Hong WK: Biomarkers as intermediate end points in chemoprevention trials. JNCI 1990 (82):555-560

11 Steel M, Thompson A, Clayton J: Genetic aspects of breast cancer. Br Med Bull 1991 (47):504-518

12 Houlston RS, Murday V, Harocopos C, Williams CB, Slack J: Screening and genetic counselling for relatives of patients with colorectal cancer in a family cancer clinic. Br Med J 1990 (301):366-368

13 Fentiman LS: Breast cancer prevention with tamoxifen. Eur J Cancer 1990 (26):655-656

14 Powles TJ, Hardy JR, Ashley SE et al: A pilot trial to evaluate the acute toxicity and feasability of tamoxifen for prevention of breast cancer. Br J Cancer 1989 (60):126-131

15 Lippman SM and Hong WK: Second malignant tumors in head and neck squamous cell carcinoma: the overshadowing threat for patients with early-stage disease. Int J Rad Oncol Biol Phys 1989 (17):691-694

Familial Cancer Control

Cancer Prevention Through Genetic Counselling

Hansjakob Müller

Research Group of Human Genetics, Department of Research, Kantonsspital, Basel, Switzerland

Several types of familial cancer can be prevented from progressing to advanced stages by regular surveillance of the person at risk [1] and hence by the early treatment of the developing neoplasia. Genetic counselling of such patients and their relatives is, therefore, an important task which often remains unrecognised. This is especially true for the common familial forms of cancer such as breast and colorectal cancer which aggregate in the families of about 5% of all patients according to the rules of autosomal-dominant inheritance [2]. The prevention of cancer is promising, especially for the familial forms because persons at risk are motivated to take preventive measures, in particular when they can be identified with certainty and counselled with concrete information [3].

The main considerations involved in the process of genetic counselling [3] and aspects specific to cancer are listed in Table 1.

An accurate diagnosis of a genetic trait is a prerequisite for informative and reliable genetic counselling. This objective can be easily achieved in rare disorders such as the hamartoma syndromes (neurofibromatosis I,

Table 1. Genetic counselling - aspects specific to cancer

Elements of genetic counselling	Aspects specific to cancer
1. Accurate diagnosis of a genetic disease or a predisposition	- Heterogeneity - Reduced life expectancy - Late manifestation - Variable expressivity and penetrance
2. Determination of genetic risk (recurrence)	- Difficult to assess
3. Communication of genetic and medical facts to the counsellee	- Many disciplines involved - Acceptance of information and advice by both patients and physicians
4. Evaluation of possible options and alternatives for dealing with a genetic burden	- Associated tumours (Which cancer to screen for and how often?)
5. Follow-up and continuing support of the counsellee and his/her family	- Change of family doctor and familial relations

von Hippel-Lindau syndrome, tuberous sclerosis, Cowden's syndrome or basal cell naevus syndrome) which show unequivocal clinical symptoms. The situation is different in other susceptibilities where cancer is the main or single manifestation. In this instance, systematic pedigree analysis remains the sole possibility for disease recognition, although it often gives only limited information. In general, women are better informed about their families and thus more information is available concerning relatives on the maternal than on the paternal side. With the exception of childhood malignancies, familial cancer develops later in life so that persons (including relatives) at risk may still be healthy. Since only a small proportion of common cancers in the general population are assumed to result from a susceptibility, this leads also to the observation of families with many sporadic cases. Unequivocal identification of the underlying genetic trait is especially difficult in familial associations of different forms of malignancies such as the cancer family-syndrome or the Li-Fraumeni-syndrome [4]. In addition, several observations related to familial breast, colorectal and other cancers point to heterogeneity of the underlying predispositions and/or variable penetrance and expressivity of the underlying traits [2]. Therefore, reliable assessment of genetic cancer risks for relatives is often very difficult. This situation may change in the near future thanks to the close collaboration between genetic epidemiologists and molecular geneticists, resulting in the unequivocal identification of the genes in question and their mutations.

Genetic counselling is a multifaceted process and involves more than an accurate diagnosis and risk estimate. The counsellee expects and deserves an open and reasonable answer to his questions about the implications of this disposition or his family history. The possible options for dealing with the genetic burden will be evaluated in several other contributions in this volume. In the discussion with the counsellee problems may develop due to the often unusual number of medical professionals involved, who hold many different views.

The family doctor is the key person in the management of the patient and in the interaction between specialised clinicians, medical geneticists, laboratory scientists and others. However, it is often a difficult, if not impossible task for him to follow individual patients and their relatives regularly and, especially, to reach extended families. For this reason, the establishment of national or regional registries for familial cancer has to be promoted to improve the follow-up and continuing support of the counsellee and his/her family. Recall of patients and relatives can easily be organised by such institutions in close collaboration with the doctors concerned. They are also helpful in providing information about new findings on the diagnosis and care of a particular familial cancer. Registries turn out to be very useful for the long-term storage of important genetic data, so that even when a change of family doctor or clinician takes place or if family relations are interrupted, for instance by divorce, there is continuity in follow-up.

REFERENCES

1 Müller Hj and Vasen HFA: Prävention familiärer Tumorkrankheiten durch genetische Beratung und Frühdiagnostik. Schweiz Med Wschr 1990 (120):1451-1460

2 Müller Hj: Dominant inheritance of human cancer. Anticancer Res 1990 (10):505-512

3 Müller Hj: Genetic counselling and cancer. In: Weber W, Laffer UT, Dürig M (eds) Hereditary Cancer and Preventive Surgery. Karger, Basel 1990 pp 12-18

4 Müller Hj: Familial cancer in Basel: some aspects. In: Müller Hj, Weber W (eds) Familial Cancer. Karger, Basel 1985 pp 1-5

Identification of Persons at High Risk for Cancer: A Delay in UV-Induced DNA Repair is Correlated with Multiple Skin Cancer

M. Roth [1], Hj. Müller [1], U.W. Schnyder [2], F. Pelloni [2], J.M. Boyle [3] and C. Sigg [2]

1 Laboratory of Human Genetics and Department of Research, Univeristy Clinics, Kantonsspital Basel, Switzerland

2 Department of Dermatology, University Hospital of Zürich, Switzerland

3 Department of Biochemical Genetics, Paterson Institute for Cancer Research, Christie Hospital and Holt Radium Institute, Manchester, United Kingdom

Solar radiation has been implicated as a possible cause for the rising world-wide incidence of malignant melanoma (MM) [1-6]. Other, additional effects may be: a) changes in social behaviour that lead to a greater exposure to sunlight, and b) the increasing penetration of UV light [7]. Xeroderma pigmentosum (XP) has been used as a model to study the possible relationship between inadequate DNA repair and the development of different types of skin tumours [8-12]. Other investigators studied the causal relationship between the above-mentioned factors and MM, the dysplastic naevus syndrome (DNS) and other forms of skin tumours [3,7,11-24]. The role of UV light in the development of DNS and MM has not been elucidated as yet. DNS is assumed to be a precursor of MM, since it is observed frequently in association with familial melanoma [12-32]. Genetic studies have provided evidence for a significant correlation based on the occurrence of both diseases in single individuals and families [14-25].

In an earlier study, using a monoclonal antibody that is specific for thymine-thymine (T-T) dimers, we found that UV-induced DNA repair was associated with a rapid loss of T-T dimer antigenicity in the cells of normal individuals, but was reduced in 20 patients with MM and in 14 DNS patients [31].

Subsequent to this study we investigated 30 patients suffering from MM, 11 patients with DNS and 20 probands who had to undergo skin biopsies for other clinical reasons.Two sets of data are presented here. In the first set, we compare the UV-induced immunokinetics of the 3 groups: MM, DNS and controls. In the second set, we compare patients suffering from a single malignancy to those who developed multiple skin tumours in each of the 2 skin cancer groups.

The results suggest a correlation between multiple skin cancer and a delay in UV-C induced DNA repair, which cannot be explained yet. Further studies investigating the induction of DNA-repair genes and the inheritance of DNA-repair defects in relation to different forms of skin cancer have to be carried out. In addition, one has to consider the delay in DNA repair as the manifestation of a more general defect of cell metabolism in multiple cancer.

Material and Methods

Probands and Skin Biopsies

The probands were chosen by 2 members of our team (C. Sigg and F. Pelloni, Department of Dermatology, University Hospital Zürich, Switzerland); skin biopsies were coded with running numbers.

The history of the disease, the family history, age, sex, skin colour, hair colour and sun exposure were documented for each proband.

After determination of the individual repair kinetics as described above, the cancer patients were identified and grouped.

Fibroblasts and UV-C Radiation

Fibroblasts were generated from skin biopsies as described previously [33] and cultivated in minimal essential medium (MEM) supplemented with 10% foetal calf serum (Gibco), 8 mM L-glutamine (Gibco) and 1% MEM-vitamine mix (Gibco).
Fibroblasts were used for the assay between passage 3-5. Confluent cell cultures were irradiated with 10 Joule/m^2 (UV-C, 254 nm, Phillips, 6V germicidal lamp, 0.2 J/m^2/sec). Fresh growth medium was added and the cells were incubated at 37°C for various additional lengths of time: 0, 10, 30, 60, 90 and 120 minutes. The cultures were allowed to recover under normal culture conditions for 10, 30, 60, 90 and 120 minutes, followed by freezing. All experiments were done in triplicate [33].

DNA Extraction and ELISA

DNA was extracted and quantified at 260 and 280 nm [34] and loss of antigenicity was determined by ELISA [33]. Triplicate assays of each sample were performed for each time point.

Statistics

The Mann-Whitney U-test was used to compare the loss of antigenicity of the controls with each of the other groups.
Variance analysis was done by the F-test to compare the frequency distribution of the subgroups (single or multiple cancer) within each of the 2 skin cancer groups (MM, DNS) and compared to the healthy controls.

Results

Loss of Antigenicity During Two Hours Following UV-C Irradiation

Figure 1a shows the loss of antigenicity in all patients suffering from MM during 120 minutes after the fibroblasts were irradiated with 10 J/m^2 UV-C light. Compared to healthy controls, the MM-patients had a significantly lower loss of antigenicity at all time points after 10 minutes ($p<0.04$; U-test). The variance was approximately 2 times higher in MM patients than in healthy controls.

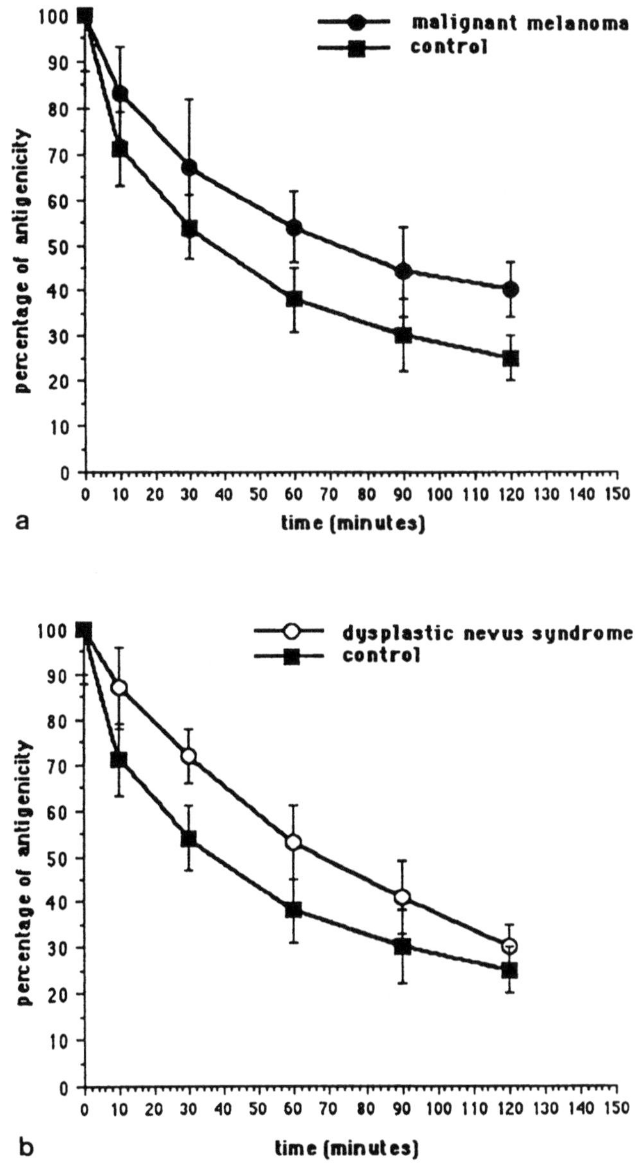

Fig. 1. Kinetics of the loss of antigenicity in patients suffering from malignant melanoma (1a) and patients suffering from dysplastic naevus syndrome (1b) compared to healthy controls. Each data point represents the mean ± S.D. of all investigated individuals of each group

Table 1. Mean ± SD for malignant melanoma, dysplastic naevus syndrome and healthy controls at each investigated time point

		Minutes after UV-irradiation				
	n	10	30	60	90	120
Controls	20	72 ± 7	51 ± 6	36 ± 4	28 ± 4	20 ± 3
MM	30	81 ± 2	67 ± 10	54 ± 11	45 ± 9	38 ± 12
DNS	11	87 ± 7	70 ± 9	50 ± 9	42 ± 8	24 ± 5

The DNS patients showed statistically significant differences at time points 10, 30 and 60 minutes after UV-C irradiation (Fig. 1b) compared to controls ($p < 0.01$; $p = 0.02$; $p = 0.05$; U-test). This effect is opposite to that observed in MM patients, who became different at later time points. The variance in the DNS patients was not as great as that observed in the MM group.
Means and standard deviations of all 3 groups, at each time point, are presented in Table 1.

Loss of Antigenicity in the Three Skin Cancer Groups

We subdivided the patients within each cancer group into those who developed a single skin tumour (s) and those who suffered from multiple skin tumours (m). The subgroups of each group were compared within the group and compared to the healthy controls at each investigated time point by the U-test (Table 2).
The frequency distribution of the MM patients is shown in Figure 2a and 2b at time points 30 minutes and 60 minutes after UV irradiation. The distribution pattern of the 2 subgroups changes with time. Within the MM group the 2 subgroups showed different kinetics of the loss of antigenicity. Compared to healthy controls the patients suffering from a sMM show a reduced loss of antigenicity, but the difference is not significant. In contrast, the patients suffering from mMM show a significant delay in the loss of antigenicity during the observed time period (Table 2). No significant differences between the 2 subgroups were observed for the onset of the disease.
Comparing the 2 subgroups of the DNS patients to the healthy controls we observed significantly different frequency distributions for both subgroups (Table 2) at the early time points (10-60 min; Figure 3a and 3b). Interestingly, the loss of antigenicity observed in the sDNS subgroup reached the level of the healthy controls after 90 minutes of repair whereas the mDNS-subgroup remained reduced for the observed time course (Table 2). Comparing the age of onset in both subgroups we observed no significant differences.

Table 2. P-values calculated by the Mann-Whitney U-test for homogeneity of skin cancer subgroups and healthy controls at each investigated time point

	Minutes after UV-C irradition				
	10	30	60	90	120
mMM/sMM	0.05	0.02	0.01	0.01	0.01
mMM/control	0.05	0.01	0.005	0.001	0.001
sMM/control	0.10	0.12	0.08	0.15	0.15
mDNS/sDNS	0.02	0.02	0.04	0.04	0.05
mDNS/control	0.001	0.005	0.01	0.01	0.02
sDNS/control	0.01	0.02	0.04	0.07	0.25

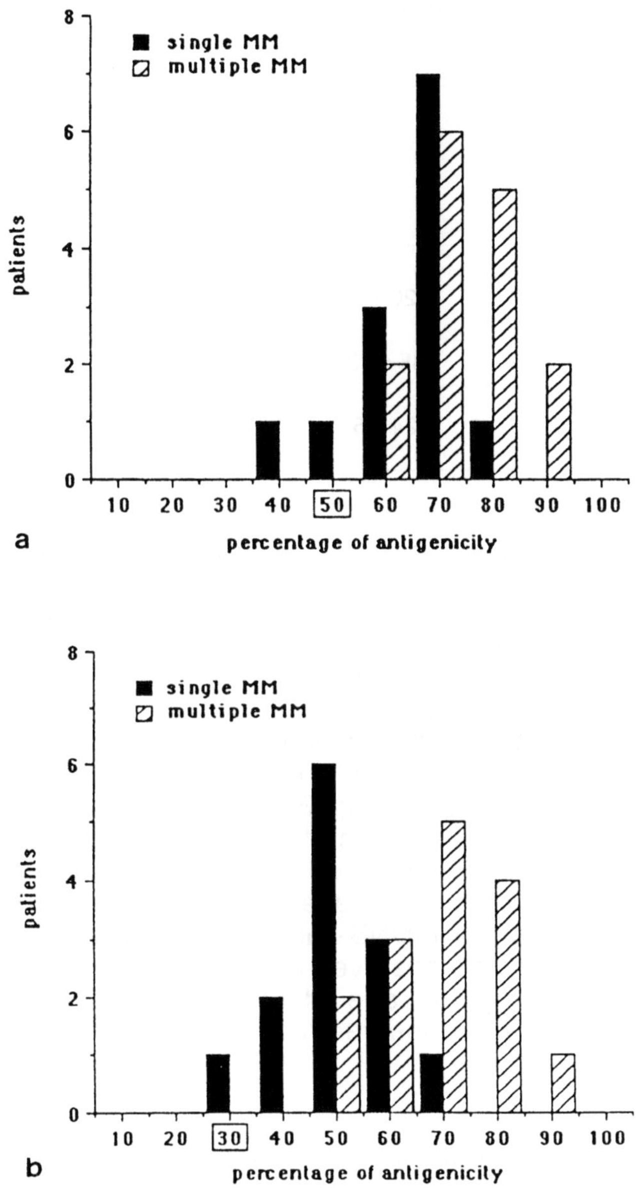

Fig. 2. Frequency distribution of the 2 subgroups of patients suffering from malignant melanoma at time points 30 (2a) and 60 minutes (2b) after UV irradiation. Indicated values (loss of antigenicity) represent the mean of the healthy controls

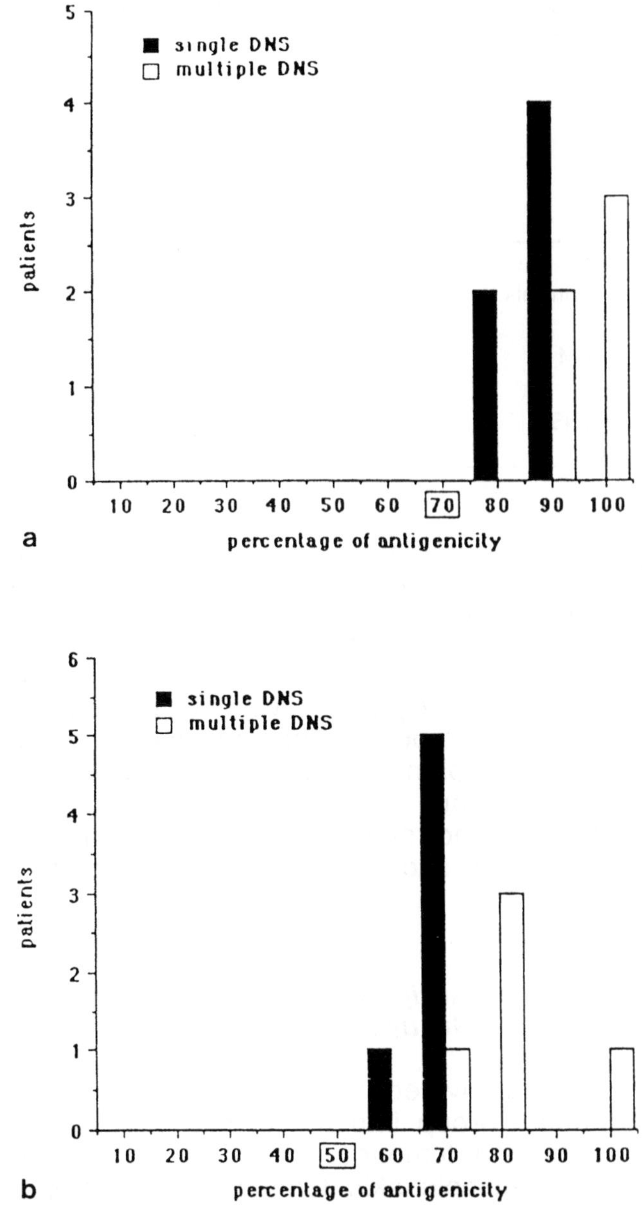

Fig. 3. Frequency distribution of the 2 subgroups of patients suffering from dysplastic naevus syndrome at time points 10 (3a) and 30 minutes (3b) after UV irradiation. Indicated values (loss of antigenicity) represent the mean of the healthy controls

Discussion

There seems to be a deficiency in the DNA-repair process in DNS and MM patients [10,12,14-21,23,31,32], which has not yet been resolved in more detail. From our earlier studies [31,33] and the present results we concluded that the DNA-repair deficiency in both cancer groups is different, since melanoma patients had delayed repair kinetics at later time points compared to DNS patients. As shown earlier, at least one-third of the MM patients showed similar repair kinetics as were observed in DNS patients [31]. These findings were supported by our new data, where individual repair kinetics were analysed (data not shown). We conjecture that there are different subgroups within each pool of patients which we cannot identify by the usual diagnostic methods.

Recent studies have disclosed that DNS and melanoma patients have unique genes that are hypermutable following exposure to UV light or to UV-mimetic chemicals [14-19]. Lymphocytes and fibroblasts from XP, melanoma and DNS patients have an increased UV-induced chromosomal instability [17,20, 32].

Possibly, dysplastic naevi have a genetic predisposition for being transformed into a melanoma by a single or perhaps a few additional events [7,16,18,20,25,32,35]. Sunlight has been alleged to be one of the major risk factors for the development of single or multiple MM [1-22]. Additional factors may be involved: hypersensitivity to sunlight [12-16], repeated sunburn during childhood [2,4,36,37], prolonged exposure to sunlight [2,9,19,36-38], and a genetic predisposition to melanoma [11,12,15-18,21,36-39]. Genetic predisposition may be due to a somatic deletion or to inactivation of protective genes, as was observed in an animal model [41]. Ananthaswamy and Pierceall [42] recently described similar molecular mechanisms of UV light in carcinogenesis in man. The authors observed activation of the ras-oncogene in human skin cancers by mutation. Most of the mutations were localised in pyrimidine-rich sequences, which have been identified as a target for UV-induced DNA damage. Similar findings have been reported by others [6,23,24,42,49].

The results presented in the second part of the study point to different reduced kinetics of the repair of UV-induced thymidine dimers in patients suffering from multiple forms of skin cancer, both mMM and mDNS. It has been suggested that UV-induced DNA damage can lead to: a) changes in the structure of chromatin [23,24,44,46,47,49]; b) generation of multiple gene copies [42,47] and c) induction of specific repair complexes [42-49]. The links between carcinogenesis and changes of the chromatin structure have been discussed in detail by Boulikas [48] and Marusic [50]. From our data we can only suggest that skin fibroblasts obtained from patients suffering from multiple forms of skin cancer lost part of their ability to repair UV-induced DNA damage; these findings might be explained by an overall reduced cell metabolism, or by changes of specific genes.

Since cancers do not arise immediately after a single exposure to physical or chemical carcinogens, the involved oncogenes may remain latent for some time, until a second event triggers further tumour progression into more malignant stages. Such additional events involve activation of other oncogenes [44,46-48], deletion of suppressor genes [41], amplification of proto-oncogenes [42,47], and other as yet unkown events. A few studies discuss the involvement of oncogenes in UV carcinogenesis [44,46-48], while the role of tumour suppressor genes in UV carcinogenesis is unknown.

One can speculate that DNA-repair enzymes would confer susceptibility to both spontaneous and environment-induced cancer. Another potential factor which can function as a tumour suppressor gene is the normal c-Ha-ras gene [42], which suppresses transformation by mutated ras gene [49].

From our earlier observations [31] we realised the importance of tracing those DNS patients who express atypical DNA repair kinetics but who have not yet developed a melanoma. It may be possible to identify individuals at high risk of developing a melanoma with a "repair" assay before the disease has commenced. Thus we would be able to recommend strategies that would minimise the environmental factors promoting the carcinogenesis of a melanoma. Such studies would also provide new insights into the aetiology of the disease.

REFERENCES

1 Lancaster HO: Sun light as a cause of melanoma. A denial survey. Med J Aust 1957 (1):452

2 Anaise D, Steinitz R and Hur NB: Solar radiation: A possible etiological factor in malignant melanoma in Israel: A retrospective study (1960-1972). Cancer 1978 (42):299-304

3 Teppo L, Pakkanen M and Hakulinen T: Sunlight as a risk factor of malignant melanoma of the skin: Cancer 1978 (14):2018-2027

4 Lee JAH: Sunlight and the etiology of malignant melanoma. In: McCarthy WH (ed) Melanoma and Skin cancer. Proceedings of the International Cancer Conference, Sydney 1972, Sydney VCN Blight 1972 pp 83-94

5 Loggie BW and Eddy JA: Solar considerations in the development of cutaneous melanoma. Semin Oncol 1988 (15):494-499

6 MacKie RM: Risk factors, diagnosis, and detection of melanoma. Curr Opin Oncol 1991 (3):360-363

7 Elwood JM, Lee JAH and Walter SD: Relationship of melanoma and other skin cancer mortality to latitude and ultraviolet radiation in the United States and Canada. Int J Epidem 1974 (3):325-332

8 Cleaver JE: Defective repair replication of DNA in xeroderma pigmentosum. Nature 1968 (218):402-408

9 Robbins JH, Kraemer KH and Flaxman BA: DNA repair in tumor cells from variant form of xeroderma pigmentosum. J Invest Dermatol 1975 (64):150-155

10 Kraemer KH, Coon HG and Petinga RA: Genetic heterogeneity in xeroderma pigmentosum: Complementation groups and their relationship to DNA repair rates. Proc Natl Acad Sci 1975 (72):59-63

11 Kraemer KH, Herlyn M and Yuspa SH: Reduced DNA repair in cultured melanocytes and nevus cells from a patient with xeroderma pigmentosum. Arch Dermatol 1989 (125):263-268

12 Venema J, van Hoffen A, Karcagi V, Natarajan AT, van Zeeland AA and Mullenders LH: Xeroderma pigmentosum complementation group C remove pyrimidine dimers selectively from the transcribed strand of active genes. Mol Cell Biol 1991 (11) 4128-4134

13 Kraemer KH and Greene MH: Dysplastic nevus syndrome: familial and sporadic precursors of cutaneous melanoma. Dermatol Clin 1985 (3):225-237

14 Bale SJ, Chakravarti A and Greene MH: Cutaneous malignant melanoma and familial dysplastic nevi: evidence for autosomal dominance and pleiotropy. Am J Hum Genet 1986 (38):188-196

15 Ramsay RG, Chen P and Imray P: Familial melanoma associated with dominant ultraviolet radiation sensitivity. Cancer Res 1982 (42):2909-2912

16 Howell JN, Greene MH and Corner RC: Fibroblasts from patients with hereditary cutaneous malignant melanoma are abnormally sensitive to the mutagenic effect of simulated sunlight and 4-nitroquinoline 1-oxide. Proc Natl Acad Sci 1984 (81):1179-1183

17 Smith PJ, Greene MH and Devlin DA: Abnormal sensitivity to UV-radiation in cultured skin fibroblasts from patients with hereditary cutaneous malignant melanoma and dysplastic nevus syndrome. Int J Cancer 1982 (30):39-45

18 Perera MIR, Greene MH and Kraemer KH: Dsyplastic nevus syndrome: increased ultraviolet mutability in association with increased melanoma susceptibility. J Invest Dermatol 1983 (80):316

19 Perera MIR, Um KI and Greene MH: Hereditary dysplastic nevus syndrome: Lymphoid cell ultraviolet hypermutability in association with increased melanoma susceptibility. Cancer Res 1986 (46):1005-1009

20 Marks R, Dorevitch AP and Mason G: Do all melanomas come from "moles"? A study of the histological association between melanocytic naevi and melanoma. Austral J Dermatol 1990 (31):77-80

21 Thielmann HW, Edler L, Brukcer A and Jung EG: Fibroblasts derived from patients with dysplastic nevus syndrome are not more sensitive towards 254-nm and 312-nm ultraviolet light than fibroblasts from normal donors. J Cancer Res Clin Oncol 1991 (117):65-69

22 Tierstein AD, Grin CM, Kopf AW, Gottlieb GJ, Bart RS, Rigel DS, Friedman RJ and Levenstein MJ: Prospective follow-up for malignant melanoma in patients with atypical-mole (dysplastic nevus) syndrome. J Dermatol Surg Oncol 1991 (17):44-48

23 Takahashi H, Strutton GM and Parsons PG: Determination of proliferating fractions in malignant melanomas by anti-PCNA/cyclin monoclonal antibody. Histopathology 1991 (18):221-227

24 Hansson J, Keyse SM, Lindahl T and Wood RD: DNA excision repair in cell extracts from human cell lines exhibiting hypersensitivity to DNA-damaging agents. Cancer Res 1991 (51):3384-3390

25 Caporaso N, Greene MH and Tsai S: Cytogenetics in familial malignant melanoma and dysplastic nevus syndrome - is dysplastic nevus syndrome a chromosome instability disorder? Cancer Genet Cytogenet 1986 (2):72-78

26 Greene MH and Bale SJ: Genetic aspects of cutaneous malignant melanoma. Recent Results Cancer Res 1986 (10):45-47
27 Elder DE; Goldman LI and Goldman SC: Dsyplastic nevus syndrome: A phenotypic association of sporadic cutaneous melanoma. Cancer 1980 (46):1787-1794
28 Reimer RR, Clark WH, Greene MH and Clark WH: Precursor lesions in familial melanoma - a new genetic pre-neoplastic syndrome. J Am Med Assoc 1978 (239):744-746
29 Greene MH, Clark WH, Tucker MA and Reimer RR: The high risk of malignant melanoma in melanoma-prone families with dysplastic nevi. Ann Intern Med 1985 (15):352-356
30 Sigg C, Pelloni F and Schnyder UW: Gehäufte Mehrfachmelanome bei sporadischem und familiärem dysplastischen Nävuszellnävus-Syndrom. Der Hautarzt 1989 (40):548-552
31 Roth M, Sigg Ch and Emmons LR: Reduced ultraviolet-induced DNA repair in patients with malignant melanoma or dysplastic nevus syndrome. In: Weber W, Laffer U and Dörig M (eds) Hereditary Cancer and Preventive Surgery. Karger, Basel 1990 pp 58-66
32 Kraemer KH, Lee MM and Scotto J: DNA repair protects against cutaneous and internal neoplasia: evidence from xeroderma pigmentosum. Carcinogenesis 1984 (5):511-514
33 Roth M, Müller Hj, Boyle JM: Immunochemical determination of an initial step in thymine dimer excision repair in xeroderma pigmentosum variant fibroblasts and biopsy material from the normal population and patients with basal cell carcinoma and melanoma. Carcinogenesis 1988 (8):1203-1208
34 Maniatis T, Fritsch EF and Sambrook J. Molecular Cloning: A Laboratory Manual. Cold Spring Harbor Lab, Cold Spring Harbor, NY 1989
35 Jung EG, Bohnert E and Booren H: Dysplastic nevus syndrome: ultraviolet hypermutability confirmed in vitro by elevated sister chromatid exchanges. Dermatologica 1986 (173):297-300
36 Holman CD and Armstrong BK: Cutaneous malignant melanoma and indicators of total accumulated exposure to the sun: An analysis separating histogenic types. JNCI 1984 (73):75-82
37 Fears TR, Scotto J and Schneiderman MA: Mathematical models of age and ultraviolet effects on the incidence of skin cancer among whites in the USA. Am J Epidemiol 1977 (105):420-427
38 Green A and Siskind V: Geographical distribution of cutaneous melanoma in Queensland. Med J Aust 1983 (1):407-410
39 Green AC and O'Rourke MGE: Cutaneous malignant melanoma in association with other skin cancers. JNCI (74):977-980
40 Duggleby WF, Stoll H and Priore HL: A genetic analysis of melanoma-polygenic inheritance as a threshold trait. Am J Epidemiol 1981 (114):63-72
41 Anders A and Anders F: Etiology of cancer as studied in the platyfish-swordtail system. Biochem Biophys Acta 1978 (516):61-95
42 Ananthaswamy HN and Pierceall WE: Molecular mechanisms of ultraviolet radiation carcinogenesis. Photochem Photobiol 1990 (52):1119-1136
43 Bale SJ, Dracopoli NC and Tucker MA: Mapping the gene for hereditary cutaneous malignant melanoma-dysplastic nevus to chromosome 1p. New Engl J Med 1989 (320):1367-1372
44 Koehler DR, Awadallah SS and Glickmann RW: Sites of preferential induction of cyclobutane pyrimidine dimers in the nontranscribed strand of lacI correspond with sites of UV-induced mutation in Escherichia coli. J Biol Chem 1991 (266):11766-11773
45 Roza L, De Gruijl FR, Bergen.Henegouwen JB, Guikers K, Van Weelden H, van-der-Schans GP and Baan RA: Detection of photorepair of UV-induced thymine dimers in human epidermis by immunoflourescence microscopy. J Invest Dermatol 1991 (96):903-907
46 Hanawalt PC: Heterogeneity of DNA repair at the gene level. Mutat Res 1991 (247):203-211
47 Bianchi NO, Bianchi MS, Alitalo K and De-La-Chapelle A: UV damage and repair in the domain of the human c-myc oncogene. DNA Cell Biol 1991 (10):125-132
48 Boulikas T: Relation between carcinogenesis, chromatin structure and poly(ADP-ribosylation). Anticancer Res 1991 (11):489-527
49 Marusic M: Evolutionary and biological foundations of malignant tumors. Med Hypotheses 1991 (34):282-287
50 Hanawalt PC: Selective DNA repair in active genes. Acta Biol Hung 1990 (41):77-91

The Nurse's Role in Familial Cancer

Hans Stoll

Clinical Nurse Specialist Oncology, University Hospital, Basel, Switzerland

The aim of this paper is to define the role of the nurse in familial cancer. Such a definition is particularly difficult to make as nursing and the nurse's tasks vary according to national approaches to nursing care throughout Europe.

Theory

There is a tendency among doctors to delegate jobs that were previously done by themselves but can be done more cheaply by nurses. There is a tendency among nurses to take over doctors' tasks because it makes them feel more important. In some instances they obtain the role of "little doctors".
A better way of defining the nurse's role is to look at what nurses are trained for, or do most of the time.
This latter approach will be followed to define the nurse's role in familial cancer. The nurse's training is at the basis of this definition, which will be illustrated by the example of a pedigree of a retinoblastoma family.
Elstein et al. [1] showed in 1984 that the classic way of thinking in the medical field is that of problem solving. The so-called "problem-solving cycle" (Fig. 1) consists of the following elements:

1. Diagnosing the problem, e.g., an infection or a tumour
2. Devising a treatment plan based on research results in natural science, e.g., a chemotherapy regimen
3. Carrying out the plan, e.g., administation of chemotherapy
4. Looking back to evaluate the results, e.g., restaging, second look

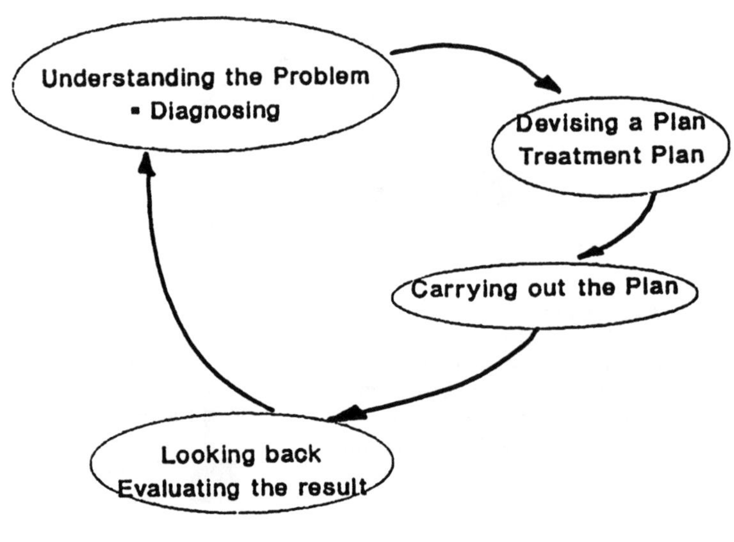

Fig. 1. Problem-solving cycle

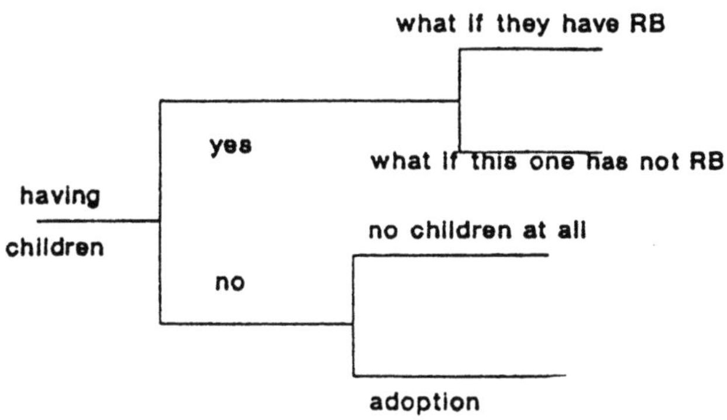

Fig. 2. Decision tree for having children when a hereditary form of retinoblastoma is present in the family

5. Returning to step 1 if the problem has not been solved (patient has not been cured or has not obtained partial remission).

The problem-solving cycle thus displays a clear starting point and a clear end point. Interestingly, the medical ethical philosopher Gillon [2] talks about dozens of decisions to be taken in ethical dilemmas but hardly at all about problems that are solved. Could it be that decision making is contradictory to problem solving?

Decision making in its true sense is never a black and white, hard and fast thing. Figure 2 shows the decision-making process by the simple example of a decision tree for a family that has to decide whether or not to have children when a hereditary form of retinoblastoma is present.

Practice

To illustrate this, the problem-solving approach and the decision-making approach are compared for the same question. Let us first have a look at the pedigree of this family (Fig. 3):

Proband's side: Sister died in an airplane crash
Father died of CML after ca-prostata

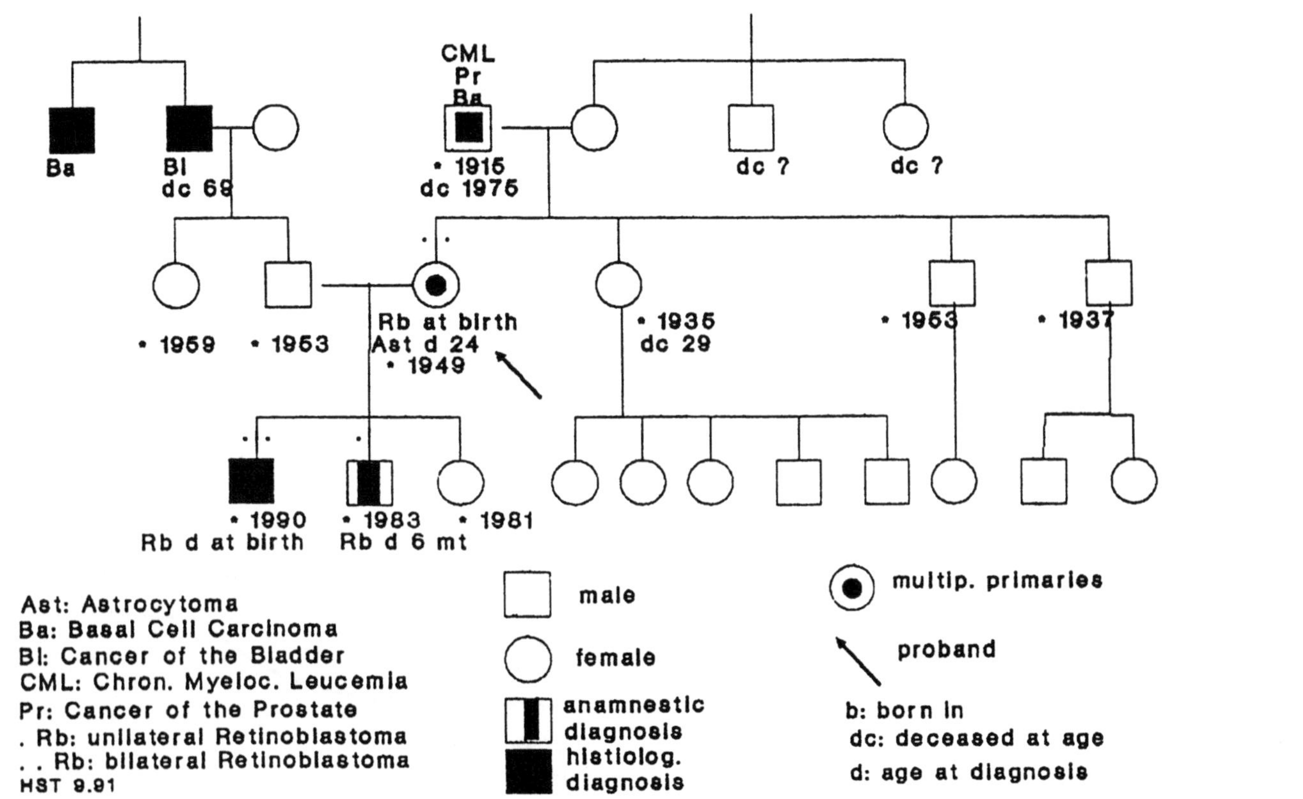

Fig. 3. Pedigree of a retinoblastoma family

Husband's side:	Father died of cardiac infarction 5 years after ca-bladder
Proband:	Had bilateral retinoblastoma diagnosed at the age of one, and the classical diagnosis of astrocytoma at the age of 24
Proband's children:	Eldest daughter no tumour First son has an anamnestically proven retinoblastoma, removed by kyosurgery Second son is born with large bilateral masses of retinoblastoma, and has a new retinoblastoma after one year.

The Problem-Solving Approach

The obvious solution of the problem of having children in a retinoblastoma family is: no children. This solves the problem of transmitting the predisposition to this type of cancer; the problem of having second primary tumours up to the age of 40; the problem of a baby having to undergo total anaesthesia every month up to the age of 3; the problem of living with a handicap and having handicapped children in this society and the problem of feelings of guilt, loss of friends, to name but a few.
Rightly, therefore, the ophthalmological clinic in Essen, Germany, says in capital letters on the leaflet provided by the medical problem solver [3]:

> "... we strongly recommend genetically predisposed people to refrain from having children."

Of course, it then says that if one decides to have children all the same, the clinic will help in every aspect (ethical insurance).

The Decision-Making Approach

If a proband considers having children, the following aspects have to be weighed against each other:
Positive:
- I live a normal life - my blindness does not bother me
- Having children for a woman means self-realisation
- There is a small chance that I do not belong to the genetically predisposed group
- Retinoblastoma can be cured in 90% of cases
- The chances of cure are improving
- I am religious, faith in God will help me
- Under no circumstances will prenatal diagnosis be carried out, abortion is no topic.

Negative:
- Problems with in-laws and friends
- Childcare is time-consuming if a child has retinoblastoma
- Additional stress/burden on the marriage if a child has retinoblastoma.

Interestingly, the problem solver's reasoning hardly applies to the proband's reasoning.
In the case of this family, the decision was to have 3 children; the third child actually had bilateral multiple retinoblastoma.

Conclusions Regarding the Role of the Nurse

Provided the medical colleagues resolve all the medical problems and assess the risk of offspring being affected by cancer, the nurse could have an important complementary role in supporting the proband in all the decisions to be taken.
Ideally, this should happen as soon as the proband starts thinking about planning a family. If both the problem-solving and the decision-making approaches are employed the patient will benefit most, suffer the least harm, receive justice and be respected in his/her autonomy [2].

REFERENCES

1 Elstein A, Shulmann L, Sprafka S: Medical Problem Solving. Harvard University Press, London 1978

2 Gillon R: Philosophical Medical Ethics. John Wiley & Sons, Chichester 1986

3 Höpping W: Parent Leaflet. Augenklinik am Klinikum Essen - Retinoblastomabteilung

4 von Winterfeldt D, Edwards W: Decision Analysis and Behavioral Research. Cambridge University Press 1986

Screening for Colorectal Neoplasia in Families

B.M. Stephenson [1,2], V.A. Murday [2], P.J. Finan [1] and D.T. Bishop [2]

1 Department of Surgery, Leeds General Infirmary
2 Imperial Cancer Research Fund, Genetic Epidemiology Laboratory, University of Leeds, Leeds, United Kingdom

Apart from age, a family history of colorectal cancer represents the single most important risk factor for developing colorectal neoplasia, with first-degree relatives of patients with colorectal cancer having a 2-3 fold increased risk [1]. These individuals represent a group who can be targeted for screening. Compliance is likely to be high and more invasive screening techniques acceptable. However, finding these relatives (○) (Fig. 1) within the population requires taking family histories from everyone (● , ○ and ◍). One solution to this is to take family histories from those individuals with colorectal cancer (●), quickly identifying those at risk within the population (○) but requiring very little work in terms of collecting family trees. As the diagnosis of colorectal cancer is established without doubt in the index case, this avoids the need for verifying a reported family history of colorectal cancer which would otherwise be necessary if relatives were accrued in other ways.

We therefore decided to look at the feasibility of screening the first-degree relatives of patients treated for colorectal cancer by one author (PJF) between 1987-1991. The idea was to see if a colorectal surgeon or gastroenterologist could practically take on the screening of individuals identified in this way. The family history of a deceased patient was obtained from the spouse. Individuals with one affected relative and aged between 50 and 75 years of age were screened by faecal occult blood test (Haemoccult ®) and flexible sigmoidoscopy. Individuals aged 50-75 years with 2 or more affected relatives were screened by faecal occult blood tests and colonoscopy. If there were 3 or more affected members in a family, colonoscopic screening was offered from age 35. Colonoscopic screening was also offered to the relatives of patients diagnosed below the age of 45, those with a positive faecal occult blood test, or adenomas on sigmoidoscopy.

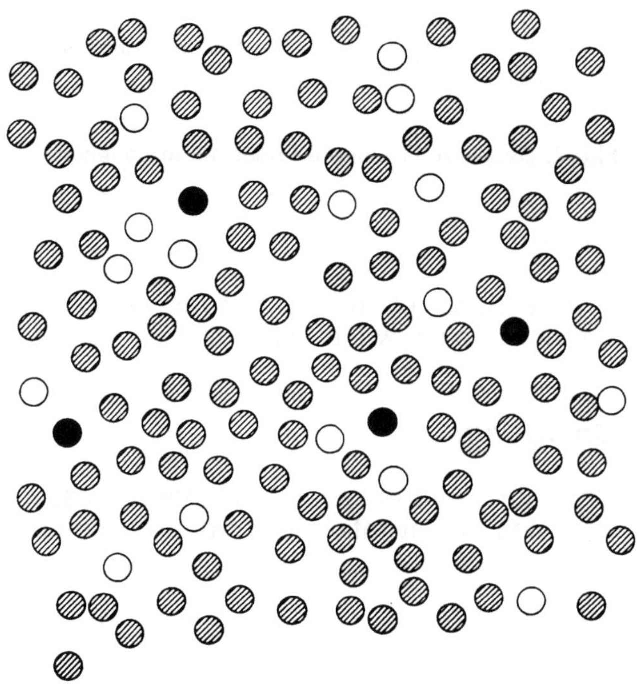

Fig. 1. Identifying the risk of colorectal cancer within the population
● = patients with colorectal cancer; ○ = relatives at risk; ◍ = others

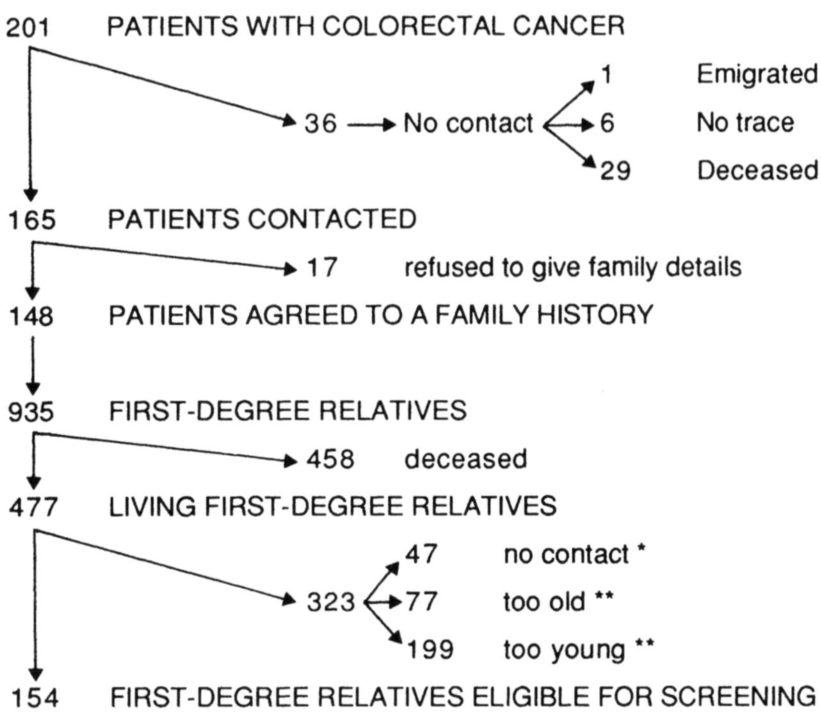

* these relatives were overseas, had lost touch with the index case or we were asked not to make contact
** as defined by screening protocol

Fig. 2. Details of first-degree relatives of patients

Results

A breakdown of those relatives eligible for screening is shown in Figure 2.

Compliance

One hundred and seven first-degree relatives accepted the invitation for screening (compliance 69%) as compared to 30 of 64 spouses (47%) (x2=19.4, $p < 0.001$). The method of endoscopic screening did not affect compliance (x2=0.02, $p > 0.5$). Older relatives and spouses were less likely to comply as were males compared to females (Table 1). Relatives of deceased index cases were more likely to comply with screening (83%) as compared to those of index cases still alive (66%) (x2=4.9, $p < 0.05$).

Table 1. Compliance for endoscopic screening

	Relatives (%)	Spouses (%)	
Overall	69	47	(p < 0.001)
Sex			
Male	65	44	(p < 0.01)
Female	73	48	(p < 0.001)
Age (years)			
< 50	100	100	(N/S)
50-60	80	44	(p < 0.001)
> 60	54	38	(p < 0.05)

Faecal Occult Blood Testing

Faecal occult blood tests were completed in all screened individuals. Three were positive: one in a female relative aged 73 and two in female spouses aged 60 and 67.

Endoscopy and Pathology

Fifteen of the 107 relatives wished to be screened at their local hospital. Ninety-two relatives attended this hospital for screening with some travelling over 200 miles.

Seventy-one individuals (mean age 58, range 50 to 74) with a single affected relative and 28 spouses (mean age 56, range 43 to 74) underwent flexible sigmoidoscopy with one relative and two spouses examined by colonoscopy. Flexible sigmoidoscopy was completed to the junction of the sigmoid and descending colon in all patients. Twelve first-degree relatives and 3 spouses had adenomatous polyps ($x2=1.5$, $p >0.10$). The mean size of the adenomas was 0.9 cm in relatives and 0.7 cm in spouses. Three relatives had 2 or more adenomas on sigmoidoscopy. The 3 spouses had subsequent normal colonoscopies whereas one relative had a further adenomatous polyp (1 cm) in the mid transverse colon.

Twenty individuals (mean age 56, range 38 to 71) with 2 or more affected relatives or a relative aged less than 45 underwent colonoscopy as their primary investigation. In 17 of these relatives flexible sigmoidoscopy was performed after sedation and before colonoscopy to estimate the false-negative rate had only flexible sigmoidoscopy been used. Two relatives (10%), both aged 42, had 2 adenomatous polyps (1 and 1.5 cm), one of which was caecal and would have been missed by flexible sigmoidoscopy (Table 2). In addition, one further relative had a large (2 cm) hamartomatous polyp in the distal transverse colon [2].

A further 20 relatives (mean 46 years, range 33-49) who were not eligible for screening by this protocol, asked to be screened. All had only a single affected first-degree relative. One male aged 45 with a positive faecal occult blood test underwent colonoscopy and was found to have a 1.5 cm moderately dysplastic adenoma at 20 cm. The other 19 relatives had normal sigmoidoscopies.

Faecal occult blood tests were unhelpful in predicting the presence of adenomas. Of those found at endoscopy only one was detected by faecal occult blood testing. In individuals to be screened by flexible sigmoidoscopy, the 3 positive faecal occult blood tests led to unnecessary colonoscopies. Two colorectal cancers are known to have occurred during the period of this study: one in a non-compliant individual with 2 affected first-degree relatives, and one in a relative aged 76 whose daughter developed colorectal cancer at 42 years of age. No cancers have occurred in the 64 spouses.

Discussion

Flexible sigmoidoscopy is a sensitive method of detecting colorectal neoplasia distal to the splenic flexure, an area which harbours over 75% of all adenomas and 90% of adenomas more than 1 cm in size [3]. The examination is quickly and easily performed without the need for full bowel preparation and results in little patient discomfort [4,5]. In contrast to 2-yearly screening by faecal occult blood tests with an observed fall in compliance [6], examination by flexible sigmoidoscopy may need

Table 2. Yield of colorectal adenomas by flexible sigmoidoscopy

	Adenoma yield	Mean size	Mean age
One affected relative (n=72)	12 (17%)	0.9 cm (0.5-2.5)	57
Two or more affected relatives or relative aged < 45 (n=20)	1 (5%)	1.25 cm (1.0-1.5)	42
Spouses (n=30)	3 (10%)	0.7 cm (0.5-1.0)	63

only be repeated every 5-10 years as the majority of adenomas are slow growing [7,8]. This should be performed during the period of maximum age-related risk aiming to reduce the incidence of left-sided colorectal cancer.

Our overall compliance of nearly 70% shows that this method of screening is acceptable to this group and is reinforced by the fact that some relatives were willing to travel long distances. Compliance was improved if the affected relative was dead. Interestingly, in both relatives and spouses below the age of 50 compliance was 100% and in relatives aged below 60 it was over 80%. This suggests that endoscopic screening is more acceptable to younger relatives when they perceive themselves at increased genetic risk, irrespective of its magnitude. The compliance in the spouses of our patients is similar to that attained in a population screening study using faecal occult blood tests in this country [6], suggesting that the family history was important in compliance.

If such a screening service were implemented, we estimate that one clinician would initially be offering in the range of 35-40 flexible sigmoidoscopies and 12-15 colonoscopies to the first-degree relatives of every 100 patients treated for colorectal cancer. Of those individuals being offered sigmoidoscopy, only the younger relatives would be encouraged to have a further examination perhaps 5-10 years later, thus maintaining a high compliance. Those shown to be at higher risk and requiring colonoscopy should be entered into standard 3-5 year follow-up programmes. The vast majority of those individuals too young to be offered screening had only one affected relative. Assuming 70% compliance in this group, approximately 75 individuals (for every 100 patients with colorectal cancer) remain to be screened by flexible sigmoidoscopy at a later date. Once a screening service was established, 100 patients with colorectal cancer would generate approximately 200 sigmoidoscopies in their relatives.

As about 7% of first-degree relatives undergoing screening colonoscopy will have isolated neoplasia beyond the reach of the 60 cm flexible sigmoidoscope [9], we estimate that a further 3 first-degree relatives might have been found to have adenomas. However, this extra yield would have involved a substantial increase in work-load (58 colonoscopies), in addition to the inconvience caused to these individuals, including time off work. Furthermore, cost-benefit analyses have suggested that colonoscopy would be best reserved for individuals with at least 2 or more affected relatives [10,11].

In summary, screening first-degree relatives of colorectal cancer patients by this protocol is feasible and the work-load manageable. Compliance is high and endoscopic screening readily accepted.

REFERENCES

1 Bishop DT, Burt RW: Genetic epidemiology and molecular genetics of colorectal adenomas and cancer. In: Rozen P, Reich CB, Winawer SJ (eds) Large Bowel Cancer: Policy, Prevention, Research and Treatment. Frontiers of Gastrointestinal Research. Karger AG, Basel 1991 (18):99-114

2 Murday V, Slack J: Inherited disorders associated with colorectal cancer. Cancer Surveys 1989 (8):139-157

3 Gillespie PE, Chambers TJ, Chan KW, Doronzo F, Morson BC, Williams CB: Colonic adenomas - a colonoscopy survey. Gut 1979 (20):240-245

4 Vellacott KD, Hardcastle JD: An evaluation of flexible fibreoptic sigmoidoscopy. Br Med J 1981 (283):1583-1586

5 Traul DG, Davis CB, Pollock JC, Scudamore HH: Flexible fiberoptic sigmoidoscopy - The Monroe clinic experience. A prospective study of 5000 examinations. Dis Colon Rectum 1983 (26):161-166

6 Hardcastle JD, Thomas WM, Chamberlain J, Pye G, Sheffield J, James PD, Balfour TW, Amar SS, Armitage NC, Moss SM: Randomised, controlled trial of faecal occult blood screening for colorectal cancer. Results for the first 107,349 subjects. The Lancet 1989 (i):1160-1164

7 Muto T, Bussey HJR, Morson BC: The evolution of cancer of colon and rectum. Cancer 1975 (36):2251-2270

8 Hoff G, Foerster A, Vatin MH, Sauar J, Larsen S: Epidemiology of polyps in the rectum and colon. Recovery and evaluation of unresected polyps 2 years after detection. Scand J Gastroenterol 1986 (21):853-862

9 Stephenson BM, Finan PJ, Gascoyne J, Garbett F, Murday VA, Bishop DT: Frequency of familial colorectal cancer. Br J Surg 1991 (78):1162-1166

10 Rozen P, Ron E: A cost analysis of screening methodology for family members of colorectal cancer patients. Am J Gastroenterol 1989 (84):1548-1551

11 Luchtefeld MA, Syverson D, Solfelt M, MacKeigan JM, Krystosek R, Waller J, Milsom JW: Is colonoscopic screening appropriate in asymptomatic patients with family history of colon cancer? Dis Colon Rectum 1991 (34):763-768

Risk Assessment in Hereditary Breast Cancer

Steven A. Narod

Division of Medical Genetics, Montreal General Hospital, Montreal, Quebec H3G 1A4, Canada

Breast cancer is the most common cancer in North American women [1]. Unfortunately, little is known about the environmental determinants of breast cancer; the strongest risk factors relate to reproductive and family history [2,3]. Because of the influence of family history on the risk of breast cancer, several centres now offer counselling to members of high-risk families. It is assumed that women identified to be at high risk can be followed closely with physical examination and annual mammography in order to identify developing neoplasms at the earliest possible stage. The genetic counsellor must examine a woman's family history and clinical records, and integrate information on other relevant risk factors, in order to formulate a specific risk for her of developing breast cancer within a defined period.

Risk can be defined in 2 ways: cumulative incidence refers to the probability of developing cancer during a woman's lifetime, often defined as 75 or 80 years. The incidence rate refers to the risk of developing cancer at a particular time in life, and is expressed in terms of cancers per year. The excess risk for women with a positive family history can be expressed in absolute or relative terms. In theory, we would like to know the risk for women carrying a cancer mutation, compared to non-carriers; in practice it is more common to compare the risk in relatives of breast cancer patients with that of the general population, or to relatives of healthy controls. A modest relative risk for siblings may reflect a very strong effect of a cancer gene. For example, if a susceptibility gene with a frequency of 10% in a population increases cancer risk 100-fold, the relative risk to siblings of cancer cases would only be three [4].

Incidence rates are usually calculated by dividing the number of new cancers in a population by the total number of person-years of observation. Relative risks constructed from incidence rates will be more extreme than those based on cumulative incidence. This is to be expected - a probability of 8% (the lifetime risk of breast cancer) cannot be increased 20 times. But some women carry through their lives a risk of breast cancer equivalent to 20 times the normal incidence.

Family 1816 is a large family from the United States in the Familial Cancer Registry at Creighton University, Omaha (H. Lynch, director) with 14 documented cases of breast cancer and 10 cases of ovarian cancer (2 women have both). Because a genetic marker on chromosome 17 (CMM86) has been found to be linked to cancer susceptibility in this family, it is now possible (within a reasonable degree of certainty) to identify women in this family who carry the susceptibility gene [5]. In the absence of preventive surgery, 80% of carriers will develop breast cancer by age 75, and 60% will have ovarian cancer [6]. As shown in Table 1, the lifetime relative risk of 9.1 does not adequately reflect the risk for breast cancer for the women in this family.

In most situations, gene carriers cannot be identified, and risk assessment is empiric, based on the results of case-control studies. Cancer patients are interviewed about breast cancer in their mothers, sisters, etc. These responses are compared to those of a control group of healthy women. Risk estimates are then calculated for a range of situations, e.g., one sister affected, sister and mother affected, etc. These risks are easy to understand and are readily applied to counselling. The coun-

Table 1. Estimates of relative risk (RR) for gene carriers in family 1816 vs non-carriers of the hereditary breast cancer gene

A: Calculated using cumulative incidence

	Probability of cancer to age 74		
	Carriers	Non-carriers	Relative risk
	0.80	0.088	9.1

B: Calculated using incidence rates

	Cancers per year per 1000 women		
	Carriers	Non-carriers	Relative risk
At age 40	23.0	0.60	38.3
At age 50	33.6	1.50	22.4
At age 60	50.0	2.0	25.0

sellor must decide which situation best describes the pedigree of his patient. Studies based on (relatively) small samples may lead to risk estimates which are counter-intuitive. For example, the risk assigned to sisters may be greater with an older age of diagnosis of the proband (Table 2) [7], or the cumulative risk in certain situations may approach 100% [8]. Such estimates are impractical.

Furthermore, the counsellor will be faced with several (often inconsistent) estimates of risk. Risk factors observed in the majority of epidemiological studies include: the number of relatives affected; a young age of disease onset in the affected relative; bilateral disease in the affected relative. It is also suggested that the risk to sisters of cases surpasses the risk to mothers [9]. Possible explanations for this are: the incidence of hereditary breast cancer is increasing, in keeping with the general trend; sisters may be nulliparous but mothers never are; there is a recessive component to breast cancer heritability.

Table 2. Lifetime risk of developing breast cancer for women with mother and sister affected

	Age of affected relatives		
	< 40	41-50	> 50
Epidemiologic approach [7]			
Bilateral:	18%	33%	23%
Unilateral:	25%	8%	19%
Genetic approach [13]			
Risk of carrier	39.2%	33.3%	21.6%
Lifetime penetrance	32.5%	27.6%	17.8%

Statistical analyses of breast cancer pedigrees have led most investigators to conclude that breast cancer susceptibility is best described as the dominant effect of a rare gene (frequency about 0.003) with a lifetime penetrance of roughly 80% [9-13]. There is little evidence for a residual multifactorial or polygenic component. In practical terms, this model means that a woman's lifetime risk of breast cancer is either 80% (if she is a carrier) or 4-8% (if she is not). Cases with many affected relatives are likely to be carriers, whereas those with none or few relatives with cancer are not.

If this model is valid, then the hereditary component of cancer risk can be determined by estimating the probability that a woman is a carrier, and adjusting for penetrance. Risk is then a function of family history, disease penetrance and gene frequency. Using such a model, Iselius et al. [13] predict that 40% of women developing cancer in their thirties will be carriers, compared with 10% of women presenting with cancer in their seventies. With this model, individual risks can be computed for any situation, and counselling becomes very specific. The MLINK option of the LINKAGE computer programme is well adapted to perform the calculations [14]. Limitations of the modelling approach to genetic counselling are: computer entry of data is required; it is assumed that the single-gene dominant model is correct; the risk estimates depend heavily upon the value of the gene frequency employed, a figure which varies considerably from study to study. Table 2 compares risks for a woman with a sister and mother affected, using estimates derived from the case-control study of Anderson and Badzioch [7], and from the segregation analysis of Iselius et al. [13].

A further limitation of the purely genetic model is that risk assessment will not integrate information on non-genetic factors, such as a history of benign breast disease, age of menarche and parity, or prior use of reproductive hormones. It is not yet clear how these external variables modify hereditary risk. A history of benign proliferative breast disease, in particular atypical hyperplasia, puts a woman at greater risk for developing breast cancer [15,16]. It appears that benign proliferative disease is more common in families with hereditary breast cancer, but this is not an invariable finding [17]. In several studies where the effect of family history and reproductive history were jointly assessed, a late age of menarche and high parity were protective in familial and non-familial cases [18,19]. However, if a single affected relative is sufficient for inclusion in the familial group, a large degree of mis-classification will occur as many familial clusters will be due to chance. The risk factors for these women should be the same as those for sporadic cases.

High age at first birth and low parity were risk factors for breast cancer in family 1816. Although the associations did not reach statistical significance, gene carriers with one or fewer children had 1.8 times the risk of those with two or more children and 2.3 times the risk if the age at first birth was 25 or more [6]. Studies are currently underway in this family to determine if the susceptibility to disease is associated with pre-neoplastic lesions, such as atypical hyperplasia.

REFERENCES

1 Young JL, Percy CL and Asire AJ: Surveillance, Epidemiology and End Results. Incidence and Mortality Data, 1973-1977. NCI Monogr 1981 (57):1-1082

2 Kelsey JL: A review of the epidemiology of human breast cancer. Epidemiologic Reviews 1979 (1):74-109

3 Anderson DE: Genetic study of breast cancer: identification of a high risk group. Cancer 1974 (34):1090-1097

4 Ponder BAJ: Inherited predisposition to cancer. Trends in Genetics 1990 (6):213-218

5 Narod S, Feunteun J, Lynch H, Watson P, Conway T, Lynch J and Lenoir GM: A familial breast-ovarian cancer locus on chromosome 17q12-23. Lancet 1991 (338):82-83

6 Narod SA, Lynch H, Conway T, Watson P, Feunteun J, Lynch J and Lenoir G: Decreasing age of onset in a large family with hereditary breast cancer. (submitted for publication 1991)

7 Anderson DE and Badzioch MD: Risk for familial breast cancer. Cancer 1985 (56):383-387

8 Ottman R, Pike M, King M-C and Henderson BE: Practical guide for estimating risk for familial breast cancer. Lancet 1983 (2):556-558

9 Claus EB, Risch N and Thompson DW: Genetic analysis of breast cancer in the Cancer and Steroid Hormone Study. Am J Hum Genet 1991 (48):232-242

10 Go RCP, King MC, Bailey-Wilson J, Elston RC and Lynch HT: Genetic epidemiology of breast cancer and associated cancers in high-risk families. I Segregation analysis. JNCI 1983 (71):455-461

11 Newman B, Austin MA, Lee M and King MC: Inheritance of human breast cancer: evidence for autosomal dominant transmission in high-risk families. Proc Natl Acad Sci 1988 (95):3044-3048

12 Bishop DT, Cannon-Albright L, Mclellan T, Gardner EJ and Skolnick MH: Segregation and linkage analysis of nine Utah breast cancer pedigrees. Genetic Epidemiol 1988 (5):151-169

13 Iselius L, Slack J, Littler M and Morton NE: Genetic epidemiology of breast cancer in Britain. Ann Hum Genet 1991:151-159

14 Lathrop GM and Lalouel JM: Easy calculation of lod scores and genetic risks on small computers. Am J Human Genet 1984 (36):460-465

15 Dupont WD and Page DL: Risk factors for breast cancer in women with proliferative breast disease. N Engl J Med 1985 (312):146-151

16 Carter CL, Corle DK, Micozzi MS, Schatzkin A and Taylor PR: A prospective study of the development of breast cancer in 16,992 women with benign breast disease. Am J Epidemiol 1988 (128):466-477

17 Skolnick MH, Canon-Albright LA, Goldgar DE et al: Inheritance of proliferative breast disease in breast cancer kindreds. Science 1990 (250):1715-1720

18 Brinton LA, Hoover R and Fraumeni JF: Interaction of familial and hormonal factors for breast cancer. JNCI 1982 (69):817-822

19 Anderson DE and Badzioch MD: Combined effect of family history and reproductive factors on breast cancer risk. Cancer 1989 (63):349-353

A Screening Programme for Medullary Thyroid Carcinoma and Breast Cancer for Families at High Risk

Hagal Sobol

Oncology-Genetics Unit, Centre Léon Bérard, Lyon, France

Cancer is a genetic disease. Tumour formation results from mutations at the cellular level [1]. On the other hand, numerous inherited forms of cancer have been reported [2]. Family study is an efficient means to identify genetic defects that lead to cancer. Most of the genes predisposing to rare inherited cancer syndromes have been mapped in the past 5 years [3], allowing us to identify at-risk individuals in families. The same approach can be applied to common cancers which tend to occur in familial clusters, e.g., breast carcinoma. In this article we present linkage results and a screening programme for medullary thyroid carcinoma and breast cancer.

Medullary Thyroid Carcinoma (MTC)

Familial forms of MTC are transmitted in an autosomal dominant fashion with a high penetrance. Three subgroups can be distinguished: 1) Multiple Endocrine Neoplasia type 2a or MEN-2a (MTC, pheochromocytoma, parathyroid hyperplasia); 2) MTC-only, where the adrenal tumour does not appear, and 3) MEN-2b (MTC, pheochromocytoma, marfanoid appearance, neuromas of the lips and buccal cavity, visceral ganglioneuromatosis) [4,5].

Linkage studies have localised the genetic defect predisposing to the 3 syndromes in the pericentrometric region of chromosome 10 [6-8]. The data do not suggest that different genetic loci may be at the basis of the different clinical presentations [9].

In France, the Groupe d'Etude des Tumeurs à Calcitonine (GETC) has been established to coordinate various research efforts and to advise on protocols for the screening and detection of MTC [10]. More than 110 families have been registered.

Genetic linkage provides an efficient means for detecting the carrier state of MTC prior to the onset of symptomatic disease [11,12]. As part of an ongoing programme at the International Agency for Research on Cancer (IARC), we evaluated the usefulness of 11 chromosome 10 markers (9 probes: FNRB, D10S34, D10Z1, MEN203, D10S94, RBP3, D10S15, 48-11, D10S22) [13-16] for the screening of the disease in 32 families. We analysed blood samples from 138 unaffected first-degree relatives of patients. Among these, 21 were considered to be at high risk (15%), 94 at low risk (68%). Forty-two percent of the subjects were informative with flanking markers (8 were considered to be at high risk and 40 at low risk). For the remaining patients, no probe was informative or recombinations were observed. The excess of low-risk individuals found in our series is a consequence of the large proportion of healthy subjects over 40 years old, when penetrance is nearly complete [17].

Early recognition and removal of MTC reduces the risk of subsequent metastatic disease [18]. The availability of a set of closely linked polymorphic DNA markers permits the early diagnosis of the carrier state of MTC with an acceptable degree of uncertainty. Screening efforts are focused on those at risk (pentagastrin tests). If no probe is informative (17% of the subjects in our study), screening is only based on conventional endocrine challenge. Most of the families belong to the MEN-2a or MTC-only types. The prognosis of MTC is quite similar in both subgroups. In the absence of genetic heterogeneity, the two clinical presentations are considered together for screening. In MEN-2b, the availability of only few pedigrees with more than one living case makes linkage studies difficult. Even when reduced, the restriction fragment length polymorphism (RFLP) method is precious in multiplex families, considering the poor prognosis of MTC in this syndrome.

Breast Carcinoma

Breast cancer is the most common cancer type among French women. Family history of the disease is a significant risk factor. Segretation analysis supports the existence of a major susceptibility gene, with a dominant pattern of inheritance in families with multiple affected members [19]. As for all common cancers, it is difficult to assume heredity in the case of small familial aggregations. In the absence of specific clinical and pathological features, the distinction between inherited and sporadic forms is based on a family history of the same or different neoplastic disorders, early age at onset and multiple primary tumours in individuals [20]. Several genetic diseases including breast tumours have been described [21]:

- Site-specific breast carcinoma
- Breast/ovarian cancer syndrome
- Breast cancer and gastrointestinal tract tumours
- Li-Fraumeni syndrome (breast carcinoma, sarcoma, brain tumour, haematological malignancies, adrenocortical tumours)
- Cowden's disease.

Recent studies have identified at least 2 genes predisposing to breast cancer:

1) The genes for early-onset familial breast cancer and for the breast/ovarian carcinoma syndrome have been assigned to the same locus in the chromosome 17q21 region [22,23]. Nevertheless, in some families analysis suggests genetic heterogeneity for both syndromes (i.e., several genes causing the disease) [22-24].

2) Germ-line p53 mutations (exon 7) have been found in 11 individuals from 6 families with Li-Fraumeni syndrome [25,26].

We have set up an oncology-genetics unit at the Centre Léon Bérard, with the aim of improving genetic counselling in cancer-prone families and identifying specific markers of susceptibility. This has allowed us to identify several such families and collect biological samples for molecular studies. Recruitment could be extended thanks to a French cooperative network.

In order to precisely determine gene locations, we tested 19 families with inherited breast carcinoma (14 site-specific breast cancer families and 5 breast/ovarian cancer families) with 3 chromosome 17q markers (D17S74, growth hormone, NM23) [24]. The results from preliminary analysis indicate that at least 30% of families show evidence of linkage. In a large breast cancer family, close linkage with chromosome 17 markers was excluded [26]. These results, together with previous reports, support the hypothesis of genetic heterogeneity in breast and ovarian carcinoma. Isolation of more informative markers is urgently needed and the testing of further new families will be of help to define gene location and map other susceptibility genes.

We also tested the exon 7 of 17 subjects from 12 families with features of the Li-Fraumeni syndrome, using polymerase chain reaction and direct sequencing. No mutations were found. It seems that involvement of exon 7 is not so common as previously described. The sequencing of exons 5 to 8 is in progress.

These data have important implications for the use of genetic markers in the early diagnosis of breast cancer. In breast cancer, contrary to MTC, DNA tests will not be reliable unless linkage is first independently established in the family under study. In cancer-prone families with the Li-Fraumeni syndrome, screening will be limited even if a gene has been identified, due to the wide range of tumours to be looked for. In other syndromes, before tightly linked markers or the gene itself are obtained, a family history could be of valuable help to identify breast carcinoma at an early stage.

Conclusions

The study of MTC and inherited breast carcinoma demonstrates the value of cooperative networks. Collaboration between physicians and molecular biologists is a means to understand the disease at the molecular level and to apply techniques of DNA analysis for screening.

REFERENCES

1 Weinberg RA: Oncogenes, antioncogenes and the molecular bases of multistep carcinogenesis. Cancer Res 1989 (49):3713-3721

2 Ponder BAJ: Inherited predisposition to cancer. TIG 1990 (6):213-218

3 King MC: Genetic analysis of cancer in families. Cancer Surv 1990 (3):417-435

4 Schimke RN: Genetic aspects of multiple endocrine neoplasia. Ann Rev Med 1984 (35):25-31

5 Farndon JR, Leight GS, Dilley WS, Baylin SB, Smallridge RC, Harrison TS and Wells SA: Familial medullary thyroid carcinoma without associated endocrinopathies. A distinct clinical entity. Br J Surg 1986 (73):278-281

6 Mathew CGP, Chin KS, Easton DF et al: A linked genetic marker for multiple endocrine neoplasia type 2A on chromosome 10. Nature 1987 (328):527-528

7 Narod SA, Sobol H, Nakamura Y et al: Linkage analysis of hereditary thyroid carcinoma with and without pheochromocytoma. Hum Genet 1989 (83):353-358

8 Norum RA, Lafreniere RG, O'Neal LW et al: Linkage of the multiple endocrine neoplasia type 2B gene (MEN2B) to chromosome 10 markers linked to MEN2A. Genomics 1990 (8):313-317

9 Sobol H, Narod SA, Schuffenecker I, Amos C, Esekowitz RAB, Lenoir GM and the Groupe d'Etude des Tumeurs à Calcitonine: Hereditary medullary thyroid carcinoma. Genetic analysis of three related syndromes. Henry Ford Hosp Med J 1989 (37):109-111

10 Calmettes C: Création d'un groupe d'étude des tumeurs à calcitonine. Bull Cancer 1984 (71):266-73

11 Sobol H, Salvetti A, Bonnardel C and Lenoir GM: Screening multiple endocrine neoplasia type 2A families using DNA markers. Lancet 1988 (i):62

12 Sobol H, Narod SA, Nakamura Y et al: Screening for multiple endocrine neoplasia type 2A with DNA polymorphism analysis. N Engl J Med 1989 (321):996-1001

13 Nakamura Y, Mathew CGP, Sobol H et al: Linked markers flanking the gene for multiple endocrine neoplasia type 2A. Genomics 1989 (5):199-203

14 Simpson NE and Kidd KK: Closing in on the MEN2A locus. Henry Ford Hosp Med J 1989 (37):100-105

15 Narod SA, Sobol H, Schuffenecker I, Esekowitz RAB, Lenoir GM and the Groupe d'Etude des Tumeurs à Calcitonine: Early detection of hereditary medullary thyroid cancer with polymorphic DNA probes. Henry Ford Hosp Med J 1989 (37):106-108

16 Goodfellow PJ, Myers S, Anderson LL, Brooks-Wilson AR and Simpson NE: A new DNA marker (D10S94) very tightly linked to the multiple endocrine neoplasia type 2A (MEN2A) locus. Am J Hum Genet 1990 (47):952-956

17 Easton DF, Ponder MA, Cummings T, Gagel RF, Hansen HH, Reichlin S, Tashjian AH, Telenius-Berg M, Ponder BAJ and the Cancer Research Campaign Medullary Thyroid Group: The clinical and screening age-at-onset distribution for the MEN-2 syndrome. Am J Hum Genet 1989 (44):208-215

18 Gagel RF, Tashjian AH, Cummings T et al: The clinical outcome of prospective screening for multiple endocrine neoplasia type 2A. N Engl J Med 1988 (318):478-484

19 Newman B, Austin MA, Lee M and King MC: Inheritance of human breast cancer. Evidence for autosomal dominant transmission in high-risk families. Proc Natl Acad Sci USA 1988 (85):3044-3048

20 Elston RC, Go RCP, King MC and Lynch HT: A statistical model for the study of familial breast cancer. In: Lynch HT (ed) Genetics and Breast Cancer. VN Reinhold Co, New York 1981 pp 49-64

21 Lynch HT: Genetic heterogeneity and breast cancer. Variable tumor spectra. In: Lynch HT (ed) Genetics and Breast Cancer. VN Reinhold Co, New York 1981 pp 134-173

22 Hall JM, Lee MK, Newman B et al: Linkage of early-onset familial breast cancer to chromosome 17q12-q21. Science 1990 (250):1684-1689

23 Narod SA, Feunteun J, Lynch HT et al: Familial breast-ovarian cancer locus on chromosome 17q12-q23. Lancet 1991 (338):82-83

24 Sobol H, Mazoyer S, Narod SA et al: Genetic heterogeneity of early-onset familial breast cancer. (submitted for publication)

25 Malklin D, Li FP, Strong C et al: Germ line p53 mutations in a familial syndrome of breast cancer, sarcomas and other neoplasms. Science 1990 (250):1233-1238

26 Srivasta S, Zou Z, Pirolla K, Blattner W and Chang EH: Germ-line transmission of a mutated p53 gene in a cancer-prone family with Li-Fraumeni syndrome. Nature 1990 (348):747-749

Familial Cancer Control - Report of Rapporteur

Peter A. Daly

St. James Hospital, James's Street, Dublin, Eire

Having devoted the first day of the symposium to defining the genetics, ecogenetics and epidemiologic features of familial cancer as well as the ethical issues surrounding the use of information and tissue samples from individual patients towards improving the circumstances of those at risk within the pedigree, the participants set out to decide how this information could be used towards the development of control strategies. This part of the symposium set out to explore the current status with regard to the realisation of the goal of control through the techniques available and the health carers working in the field.

Dr Roth's presentation on the identification of persons at high risk of skin cancer due to DNA repair deficiencies dealt with laboratory studies on the repair capacities of skin samples taken from patients with malignant melanoma (MM), superficial spreading melanoma (SSM) and dysplastic naevus syndrome (DNS). Control subjects attending the dermatology clinic for treatment of warts were used. Delayed repair capacity was noted mainly for patients with multiple skin malignancies in MM, SSM and DNS with some differences in timing. It could not be determined if this tendency existed prior to the development of the multiple lesions or whether it resulted from such development.

There was poor clinical data available to the laboratory markers. Further study needs to be done on families, especially with DNS, to determine if this is an inherited trait or due to environmental influences. Correlation with development of other malignancies as described earlier by Dr. Sigg would also be of interest.

The respective roles of genetic counsellors, nurses and doctors (including surgeons) were examined and discussed in detail. It was felt that the nurses' role would mainly be in supporting the proband and family with decision-making once the information had been provided by the doctor. The lack of a proper structure for Family Cancer Clinics was indicated and it seemed inappropriate to dwell on individual roles ahead of the proper overall structuring of units. If this were achieved, the development of a special discipline within the nursing profession to deal with cancer families would seem desirable. Such persons function in the U.S. at least in specialised centres and are termed "family contact persons". Patient/family support groups may also serve a useful function for cancer families but not all people desire such a service.

Dr. Müller re-emphasised the importance of gathering proper family histories and verified the reliability of anamnestic data obtained through diligent gathering of family history details. 83.5% of information was accurate and females had better recall than males with data gathered in the context of childhood cancer being most accurate due to the presence of both parents at the interview. The role of the medial geneticist in this area would seem to be the guarantee of continuity of care for the patient, the improvement of survival for family members at risk, the coordination of care for patients and family members and further advances due to the facilitation of clinical and laboratory research. The controversial subject of cancer registries was again raised and it appears that contrary to the expressed view of legislations, there is an acceptance of such a concept by patients as long as the information is used for medical purposes only. It is felt that legal action will force doctors towards obtaining family histories in sufficient detail in the future.

Much discussion took place on directive versus non-directive counselling. It seemed to be the consensus that where dogmatic information existed, counselling could be directive and it was said that patients often requested such an approach. On the other hand, where risks versus benefits could not be categorically defined it was best to provide the information in a non-directive way.

Dr. Murday reported on the feasibility of family-based screening for colorectal cancer in terms of user and provider factors. Dividing those deemed at risk into 2 groups based on the history of the index case and using the spouses as controls, she found that there was about 70% compliance, that 100 patients with colorectal cancer in the U.K. will generate 167 relatives for screening and that the overall yield was low. It did seem, however, that patients and families found the approach acceptable and that the surgeon could absorb the work generated into his practice. A number of doubts were expressed about the efficiency of the type of recruitment used.

The 2 remaining presentations in this session dealt with the use of modern laboratory techniques in the screening and estimation of risk in familial cancer. Both Drs Narod and Sobol confirmed earlier observations with regard to linkage to a gene on chromosome 17 in ductal breast cancer, showing that a 50% linkage could be demonstrated with a young age of onset and the presence of ovarian cancer making linkage more likely.

Prophylactic surgery for high-risk members of breast cancer kindreds is recommended in the early thirties. Oophorectomy can usually wait until families are completed. Attention was drawn to the development of serous surface papillary carcinoma in 3 patients in this group who had prophylactic oophorectomy, thus defining a risk for malignant transformation in other tissues of Müllerian origin. This needs to be discussed with women prior to oophorectomy which clearly does not remove the risk of malignancy completely.

A risk profile has been developed in the U.S. for use in entering patients on the NSABP Tamoxifen prophylaxis trial. This could find general use in the counselling of patients.

Dr. Sobol presented some data with regard to the p53 gene in breast cancer patients from Li-Fraumeni kindreds. This area was felt to be controversial with families described in which p53 mutations existed but with cancer cases that did not seem to have inherited the mutation.

The results in medullary carcinoma of thyroid (MTC) alone and as part of MEN-2a using probes for the centromeric region of chromosome 10 complemented by calcitonin measurements stimulated by prostaglandin as presented by Dr. Sobol, were most satisfactory as previously described in the literature. Unfortunately, live cases of MEN-2b are too few to allow application of this technology. Extensive studies in 100 families are being undertaken in France.

The major points to be taken from this session would appear to be the importance of proper family history documentation and follow-up in the clinical setting and the gap which still exists between the clinic and the application of newer molecular biology techniques in delivering clinically relevant material.

A Clinical Study of Familial Cancer in Japan

T. Nomizu [1,2], R. Abe [2], A. Tsuchiya [2], J. Utsunomiya [3], F. Watanabe [2] and Y. Yamaki [1]

1 Department of Surgery, Hoshi General Hospital, Koriyama, Japan
2 Department of Surgery II, Fukushima Medical College, Fukushima, Japan
3 Department of Surgery II, Hyogo Medical College, Hyogo, Japan

A high incidence of a particular cancer in a family points to the involvement of genetic factors. Hereditary tumours include colorectal cancer based on familial adenomatous polyposis (FAP) and medullary carcinoma of the thyroid in MEN type 2. The mode of inheritance of these cancers has been clarified. It is also known that some family lines have a high incidence of morphologically ordinary types of cancer.

This study analysed families prone to colorectal cancer, breast cancer and gastric cancer described in the Japanese literature; the aim of the study was to make a clinical characterisation of familial cancer types.

Familial Colorectal Cancer (Hereditary Non-Polyposis Colorectal Cancer, HNPCC)

Colorectal cancer is one of the cancers the onset of which seems to involve genetic factors. Two colorectal cancer-prone families are shown in Figures 1 and 2. In Japan, familial

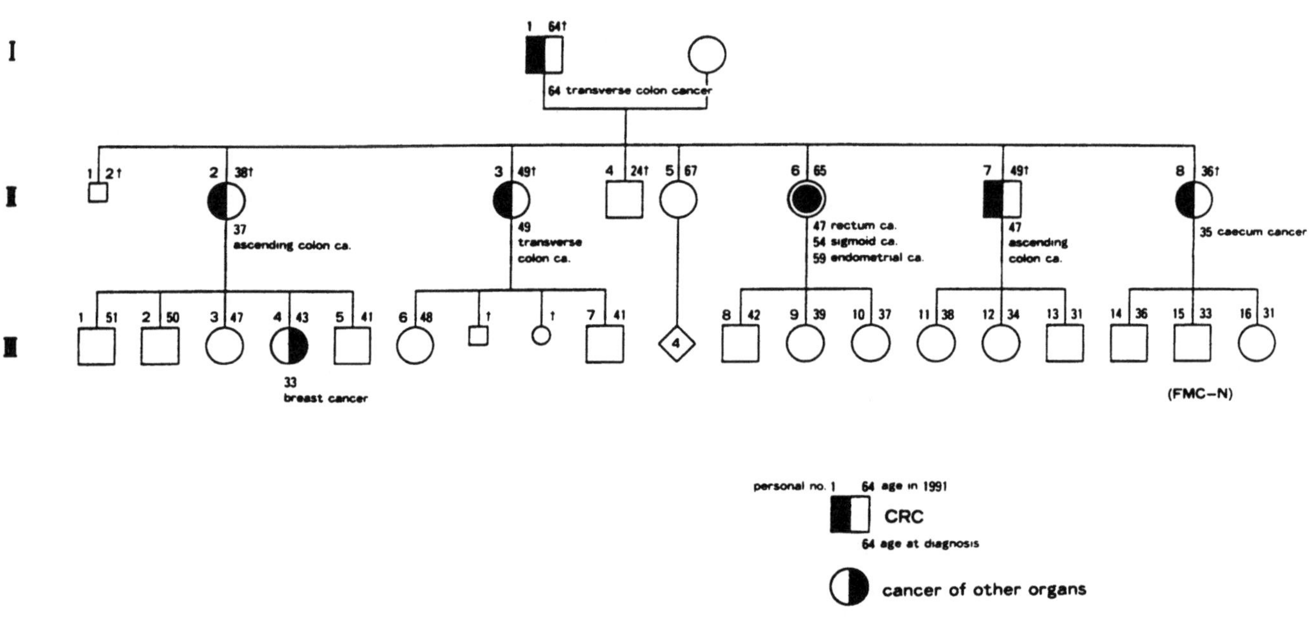

Fig. 1. Pedigree of Family 1

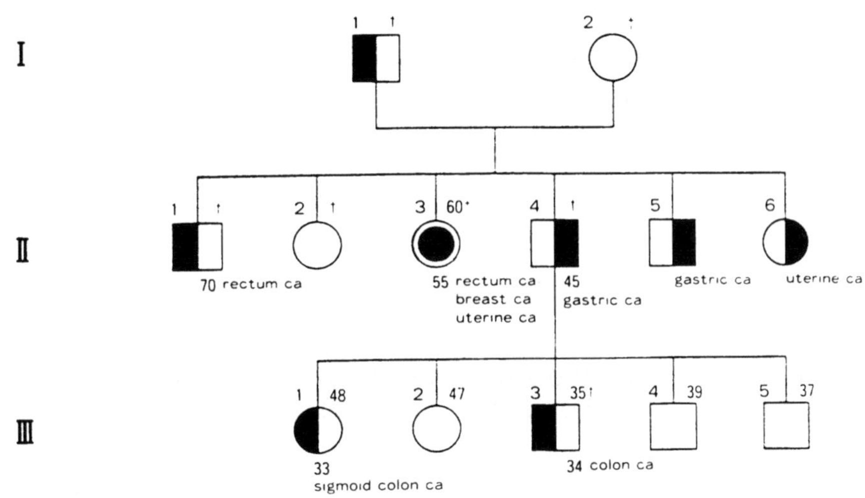

Fig. 2. Pedigree of Family 2

colorectal cancer (excluding FAP) has been reported in 49 families (219 cases) in the literature until 1991 (Table 1). We analysed the age at diagnosis, male-to-female ratio, cancer site, frequency of multiple cancers and the familial spectrum of malignant tumours in these 219 cases. One hundred and seventy-four cases of colorectal cancer without any family history of cancer served as controls (non-familial colorectal cancer group).

The age at diagnosis was analysed in 169 cases for which information was available. In cases of metachronous multiple colorectal cancer, the age at diagnosis of the first cancer was used. The percentage of colorectal cancer patients younger than 50 years of age among all cases of familial colorectal cancer was 66.4%, which was significantly higher than among controls (17.8%; $p < 0.01$). The mean age at diagnosis was significantly lower in familial colorectal cancer (44.5 years) than in controls (61.2 years, $p < 0.01$).When the mean ages were compared among the different generations with familial colorectal cancer, the mean age at diagnosis was significantly decreased by generation: 54.5 years in the first generation, 40.1 years in the second and 34.9 years in the third.

The male-to-female ratio in 179 cases of familial colorectal cancer did not differ significantly from that in the controls.

The site of colorectal cancer was analysed in 235 lesions (including multiple colorectal cancer) for which information was available. The incidence of cancer in the caecum, ascending colon, transverse colon and descending colon was higher in familial colorectal cancer than in the control group. The percentage of colonic cancer in all cases of familial colorectal cancer was 67.3%, which was significantly higher than that in the controls (45.1%; $p < 0.01$).

Of all cases of familial colorectal cancer, 28.3% had multiple cancers (multiple colorectal cancer in 14.6% and multiple cancers at different sites in 13.7%). By contrast, only 3.6% multiple cancers were seen in the control group. This difference in occurrence between the two groups was statistically significant ($p < 0.01$).

Malignant tumours other than colorectal cancer were most frequently gastric cancer (48 cases), followed by uterine cancer (33 cases, including 16 cases of endometrial cancer) in the 49 families studied (Table 1).

In conclusion, familial colorectal cancer can be characterised by an early age at onset, location predominantly in the proximal colon, and a high incidence of multiple cancers, including multiple colorectal lesions.

Familial Breast Cancer

Involvement of genetic factors is also suggested in breast cancer. In the Japanese literature familial breast cancer has been reported in 15 families so far (53 cases; Table 2). Two of these families are represented in Figures 3 and 4. The age at onset and the frequency of multiple cancers including bi-

Table 1. HNPCC IN JAPAN (Japanese criteria)

reporter	no. of families	Colorectal cancer	Gastric cancer	Duodenal cancer	Cancer of the liver & biliary tract	Breast cancer	Uterine cancer (endometrial ca)	Ovarian cancer	Lung cancer	Cancer of urinary tract	Mesenteric tumor	Brain tumor	Malignant lymphoma	Ca. of the prostata	Ca. of the skin
1. Kamegai	(1)	(4)													
2. Sasa	1	2					1								
3. Tarao	1	6	1				1								
4. Noji	1	7	1												
5. Mikawa	1	7	2												
6. Yagita	1	4				1									
7. Katano	1	5													
8. Marutani	3	20	1							1					
9. Utsunomiya	6	27	9	1			2(1)		1	1	1	2		1	
10. Ohara	1	3													
11. Koike	1	4	2												1
12. Takami	1	3	2				1(1)								
13. Sadahiro	1	4													
14. Ushio	10	34	9				10(6)	3		1			2		
15. Oshima	1	3													
16. Sasaki	1	7		1	1		2(1)		1						
17. Kouda	1	2	1		1		1(1)								
18. Igarashi	1	6					1(1)			1					
19. Tokunaga	1	9	4		3		1			1					
20. Matsuyama	2	8	1			1	2(2)								
21. Ochi	1	4	1												
22. Ishibashi	1	5					1(1)					1			
23. Kawamura	1	4					2								
24. Hiromoto	1	4	1				1			1					
25. Hanagasaki	1	6	1				1								
26. Tomoda	1	9	3		1										
27. Chiba	1	3	3				1(1)	1		5		1			
28. Ohsawa	1	4	1				2		1						
29. Nomizu	5	19	3			2	3(1)		1						
Total	49	219	46	2	6	4	33(16)	4	4	11	1	4	2	1	1

Table 2. Familial breast cancer in Japan

Reporter	No. families	breast	bilateral breast	oeso-phagus	gas-tric	colo-rectal	liver	pan-creas	thyroid	ovarian	uterine	larynx	mela-noma
Sakamoto	1	5	1	1					1		2		
Fujita	1	3	2								1		
Kasumi	4	12	6		1		1	1		2			
Koyama	1	5	2			1				1			
Sato	1	3	2		1	1							
Uchida	1	3				1						1	1
Ochiai	1	7	2										
Nomizu	5	15	1		1	1			2	1	3		
total	15	53	16	1	3	4	1	1	3	2	8	1	1

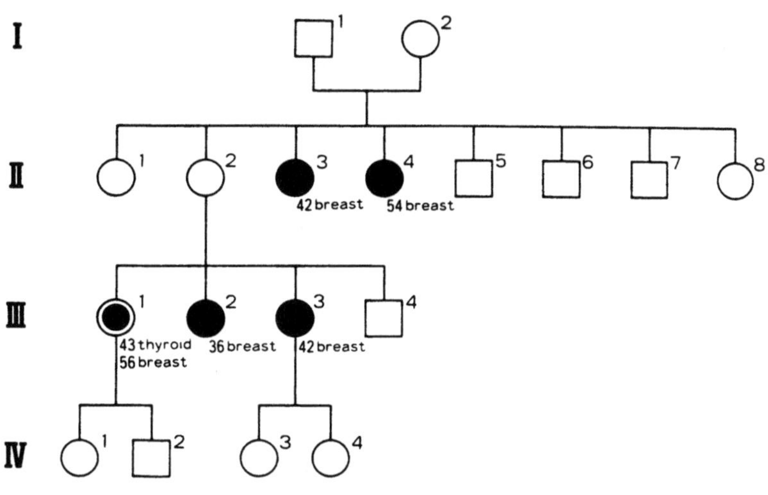

Fig. 3. Pedigree of Family 3

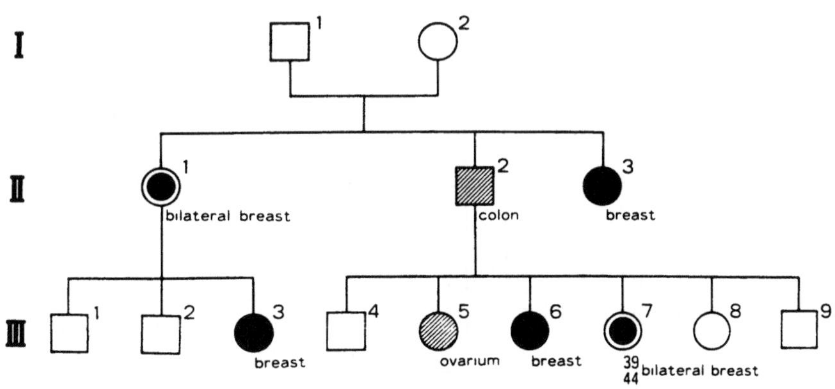

Fig. 4. Pedigree of Family 4

lateral breast cancer were analysed in these 53 cases. Two hundred and sixteen cases of breast cancer without any family history of cancer served as controls (non-familial breast cancer group).

The mean age at onset of breast cancer and the percentage of cases younger than 40 were 45.8 years and 37.0% in familial breast cancer and 50.4 years and 17.6% in the control group. Familial breast cancer tended to occur more frequently at younger ages than non-familial breast cancer.

The percentage of multiple cancers in familial breast cancer was 35.9% (30.2% bilateral breast and 5.7% in other organs). The multiple cancer rate was as low as 0.9% in the control group ($p < 0.01$).

In addition to breast cancer, the following malignant tumours were observed in these 15 families: uterine cancer in 8 cases, colorectal cancer in 4 cases, gastric cancer in 3 cases and thyroid cancer in 3 cases.

Familial breast cancer can be clinically characterised by an early age at onset and a high incidence of multiple cancers, especially bilateral breast cancer. In Japan, familial breast cancer accounted for about 5% of all cases of breast cancer.

Familial Gastric Cancer

Gastric cancer is the most frequently observed malignant tumour in Japan. However, reports on familial gastric cancer are rather scarce (50 cases from 7 families). The gastric cancer-prone families studied by us are shown in Figures 5 and 6. We analysed the age at onset, male-to-female ratio and the incidence of multiple cancers in these 50 cases, in comparison to 139 control cases of gastric cancer without any family history of cancer.

The mean age at onset of gastric cancer and the percentage of cases younger than 40 were 46.6 years and 35.4% in familial gastric cancer and 57.5 years and 5.7% in the control group. The higher occurrence of familial gastric cancer at younger ages than non-familial gastric cancer was statistically significant ($p < 0.01$).

The male-to-female ratio was approximately 1:1 in familial gastric cancer, while it was 1.3:1 in the control group. The percentage of multiple cancers did not show any significant difference between familial gastric cancer cases (4.0%) and controls (5.0%).

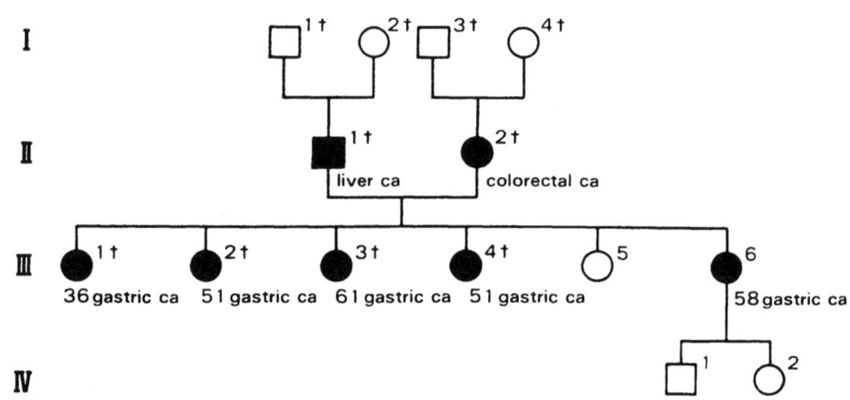

Fig. 5. Pedigree of Family 5

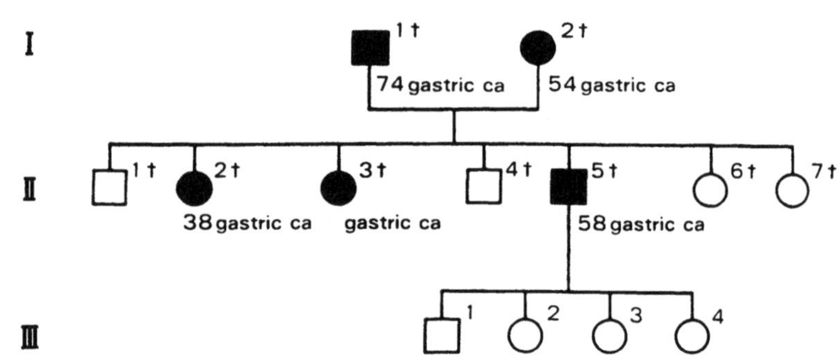

Fig. 6. Pedigree of Family 6

Thus, familial gastric cancer can be characterised by an early age at onset. The percentage of multiple cancers did not differ between the two groups.

Discussion

Familial colorectal cancer among Japanese can be clinically characterised by: 1) early age at onset and a decrease in the age at onset generation by generation; 2) predominance of cancer affecting the proximal colon, and 3) a high incidence of multiple cancers, including multiple colorectal lesions. These characteristics have also been described in previous reports [1,2]. On the basis of these findings, HNPCC in Japan can be defined as follows:

A. Three or more first-degree relatives (including the proband) have colorectal cancer.
B. Two first-degree relatives (including the proband) have colorectal cancer and one of these cases corresponds to at least one of the following criteria: a) onset of colorectal cancer at an age of less than 50; b) cancer affecting the right colon proximal from the splenic flexure; c) synchronous or metachronous multiple colorectal cancer, or d) synchronous or metachronous multiple cancers in other organs. FAP cases are excluded from this definition.

In 1991, Kunitomo et al. [3] surveyed the results of a nationally distributed questionnaire on familial colorectal cancer and analysed 777 cases of colorectal cancer using the above-mentioned criteria. The results were similar to those of the present study. Of the 49 families (219 cases) examined in the present study, 30 families (154 cases) fulfilled the criteria of the International Collaborative Group on HNPCC [4]. The analysis of cases corresponding to the ICG-HNPCC criteria also yielded results similar to those of the present study and the study of Kunitomo et al. When we analysed the spectrum of malignant tumours other than colorectal cancer in HNPCC families, gastric cancer was observed most frequently. This seems to be a characteristic of HNPCC in Japanese.

Familial breast cancer in Japanese women is characterised by an early age at onset and a high incidence of bilateral breast cancer [5]. It seems that a family history of breast cancer plays an important role in the early detection of breast cancer by mass screening. Therapeutic results have been better in breast cancer with a positive family history than in breast cancer without a family history in Japanese women, because in the former group early detection of breast cancer is more frequent than in the latter [6]. Although subtypes of familial breast cancer such as familial breast-ovarian and breast-thyroid cancer have been reported in Japan [5], these subtypes were not included in the present study. No cases of the Li-Fraumeni syndrome have been reported in Japan so far. The incidence of breast cancer in Japan has been increasing over the past decades. Breast cancer is expected to become a leading cancer among Japanese women in the 21st century. Bearing this in mind, we are planning to conduct a nationwide questionnaire survey in 1992 aimed at a more detailed clinical analysis of familial breast cancer.

Gastric cancer is the most frequent malignant tumour in Japan, with an incidence of more than 60 per 100,000 in the general population. However, reports about familial aggregation of gastric cancer are scarce, because the high incidence of gastric cancer makes it difficult to distinguish a coincidental familial aggregation of gastric cancer from a genetic one. An important characteristic of genetically determined familial gastric cancer is the early age at onset. Recent advances in molecular genetics suggest that in the near future linkage analysis will also be possible in gastric cancer.

The early age at onset is the most important characteristic of familial colorectal, breast and gastric cancer. When different generations were compared, the age at onset of these cancers in the first generation did not differ from that in cases of non-familial cancer. The early age at onset was seen in the second generation (Table 3).

Familial cancer is clinically significant in the sense that early detection and treatment are possible by screening family members for cancer. Familial cancer might provide a good model to clarify the mechanism of carcinogenesis. To allow further progress in the

Table 3. Average age of patients with familial cancer

	colorectal cancer	breast cancer	gastric cancer
Non-familial	61.2	50.4	57.5
Familial	44.5	45.8	47.6
Familial I generation	54.5	49.1	58.0
Familial II generation	40.1	40.3	41.9

study of familial cancer, we have to resolve various problems, such as: 1) establishment of a nationwide registration system for familial cancer in Japan; 2) education of physicians and associates on the importance of familial cancer; 3) problems involved in notification of cancer to patients and families; 4) cooperation among clinicians, epidemiologists, geneticists, biochemists and pathologists, and 5) social and ethical problems.

REFERENCES

1 Utsunomiya J et al: Familial large bowel cancer. In: Decosse JJ (ed) Clinical Surgery International: Large Bowel Cancer. Churchill Livingstone, New York 1981 pp 16-33

2 Nomizu T et al: Clinical investigation of familial clustering of cancer. Jpn J Cancer Clin 1986 (32):485-492 (in Japanese with English abstract)

3 Kunitomo K et al: HNPCC in Japan. In: Third Meeting of the ICG-HNPCC, and 5th International Symposium on Colorectal Cancer, Turin, Italy, September 1991

4 Vasen HFA et al: The International Collaborative Group on Hereditary Non-Polyposis Colorectal Cancer (ICG-HNPCC). Dis Colon Rectum 1991 (34):424-425

5 Nomizu T et al: Breast cancer prone family: Clinical study of familial breast cancer. Jpn J Cancer Clin 1987 (33):477-481 (in Japanese with English abstract)

6 Nomizu T et al: Clinical study of breast cancer patients with family history. Jpn J Breast Cancer 1987 (2):435-439 (in Japanese with English abstract)

DNA Diagnosis in Families with Hereditary Forms of Cancer

H.F.A. Vasen [1], Hj. Müller [2] and P. Meera Khan [3]

1 Foundation for the Detection of Hereditary Tumours, Leiden, The Netherlands
2 University Children's Hospital, Basel, Switzerland
3 Human Genetics Department, Leiden State University, Leiden, The Netherlands

Since the mid-1970s, recombinant DNA techniques have given an entirely new dimension to genetic research. For example, methods have been developed by which the coding of genes by DNA can be determined. Such developments are providing increasing information on future health, and the application of these techniques can make an important contribution to the primary and secondary prevention of disease and also provide support for family and life planning. Recently, however, concern has been expressed about possible negative social consequences of the new knowledge. The present article deals with the value of DNA analysis for application in families with a hereditary form of cancer, the implications for conventional screening, and the associated ethical issues.

Hereditary Forms of Cancer

In roughly 5 to 10% of cancer cases, genetic factors play a decisive role. The characteristics of hereditary tumours include the relatively young age at which these cancers appear and the occurrence of multiple primary tumours. The present discussion is restricted to the dominantly inherited cancer syndromes. Table 1 lists a number of dominantly inherited cancers and presents the criteria for their diagnosis.

Periodic Examination

During the last decade, mortality due to cancer has hardly declined despite improvement of the therapeutic methods. In recent years it has been realised that more attention should be paid to prevention. Periodic screening of families with a hereditary form of cancer is a form of secondary prevention and can lead to the reduction of morbidity and mortality. The benefit of screening in this high-risk group of persons is greater because of the early age at which the malignancies manifest themselves. The recommended screening procedures are shown in Table 1.

DNA Analysis in Families with a Hereditary Form of Cancer

In recent years it has become possible by means of genetic markers to trace the transmissions of the genes responsible for these diseases in families. The essential point of DNA diagnostics is to distinguish the two copies of the chromosomes the individual has. The markers allow us to follow the transmission of the genes in the affected family. An analysis based on markers has two limitations: 1) it cannot be performed in single patients: as many relatives as possible belonging to two or more generations must participate; 2) due to recombination during the formation of the sex cells, the coupling be-

Table 1. Hereditary cancers and their diagnostic criteria

Hereditary cancer	Clinical		Genetic	
	Diagnosis	Screening procedure	Location on chromosome	Accuracy of DNA diagnosis
Familial adenomatous polyposis	>100 adenomas in colon and rectum	sigmoidoscopy	5	100%
MEN-1 * syndrome	hyperparathyroidism, tumours of pancreas and pituitary	calcium, phosphate, PTH, gastrin and prolactin	11	>95%
MEN-2 * syndrome	hyperparathyroidism, medullary thyroid cancer	estimation of plasma calcitonin after stimulation, urinary catecholamines	10	100%
Neurofibromatosis (NFI)	neurofibroma, café-au-lait spots, glioma of N. opticus, pheochromocytoma	dermatological, ophthalmological and neurological examination	17	99%
Bilateral acoustic neuromas (NF2)	tumours of N. acousticus, meningioma, schwannoma	neurological examination, if necessary CT, MRI scan	22	>90%
Retinoblastoma	retinoblastoma, osteosarcoma	ophthalmological examination	13	100%
Von Hippel Lindau syndrome	retinal angioma, haemangioblastoma of the cerebellum, renal tumour, pheochromocytoma	ophthalmological and neurological examination, ultrasound, urinary catecholamines, if necessary CT, MRI scan	3	99%

* MEN syndrome = multiple endocrine neoplasia syndrome

tween marker and defective gene may be lost. The reliability of the results of a DNA analysis is determined by this chance of uncoupling. Table 1 shows the hereditary forms of cancer for which a DNA analysis is available, the chromosome in which the defective gene is located, and the maximal reliability of the results. Once the defective gene has been localised and the mutation can be demonstrated directly - as in the case of retinoblastoma - the prediction can have a reliability of 100%. Furthermore, the participation of other members of the family is no longer necessary.

Consequences of the Screening Protocol

A major advantage of linkage analysis is that after exclusion of the risk for individuals from families with genetically determined forms of cancer, the burdensome and very long-lasting screening can be avoided and the subject can be reassured. Familial adenomatous polyposis offers a good example in this respect. In this disease the patients develop hundreds of adenomatous polyps in the colon. If untreated, almost all of the patients develop colonic carcinoma. Family members who are at risk must undergo endoscopy of the colon twice yearly between the ages of 12 and 50. In these families, DNA analysis makes it possible to exclude the relevant disease gene with 100% certainty, which means that screening can be omitted [4,5].

Prenatal Diagnosis

The use of prenatal DNA linkage analysis is at present one of the possible approaches to the problem. As the hereditary forms of cancer discussed in the present paper can usually be adequately treated, if diagnosed early, it is doubtful whether this diagnostic method will be used frequently in the future.
Experience in England and Germany with familial adenomatous polyposis families has shown that there is still little demand for prenatal investigation in this group.

Ethical Aspects

The increasing availability of new diagnostic methods has made the decision much more difficult for relatives of patients and has also increased the importance of the ethical aspects of genetic counselling [6]. The relevant ethical principles are: 1) every person has the right to obtain complete information about him or herself and the right to make decisions freely; 2) all persons have the right to receive good care and assistance; 3) they are entitled to their proper share of what society has to offer; 4) the privacy of the collected data should be guaranteed.
The use of DNA analysis demands the complete agreement of the subject, who must be thoroughly informed and must be able to decide in complete freedom as to whether the possible advantages outweigh the disadvantages. Non-directive advice is the most important issue here. During the process of decision-making, the subject must be able to count on complete support. The following points must be considered when information is provided before the test is performed: 1) information must be given about the disease itself, its genetic aspects, the possibilities for treatment, and the prognosis; 2) information must be given about the tests and the need for participation of other members of the family; it must also be made clear that the results of the tests do not give any clue as to the age of onset of the disease; 3) information should be given about psychological and socio-economic consequences (insurance, employment) for the individual; 4) relatives must also be informed about sources of psychological support.
Valid guidelines for the reporting of results are: 1) results and consequences must be reported as soon as possible after the analysis has been performed; 2) relatives should retain the right not to be informed of the results; 3) ample time must be reserved for discussion of the findings; 4) the subject's general practitioner and specialist must be informed about the results as soon as possible.
DNA analysis ideally requires the collaboration of medical specialists, clinical geneticists, and, if available and necessary, the patient's association. Generally, the clinical geneticist gives the genetic information and interprets the DNA findings. Unlike the specialist in charge of the treatment, the clinical geneticist has sufficient information for optimal discussion of the often complicated and emotionally charged problems.

Social Consequences

We are all aware of the potential social consequences of genetic studies. Various authors and institutions [7] have argued for statutory regulations to protect applicants for genetic investigation against possibly damaging interests of insurers. This is not a simple problem, because misuse of the results by the subject is also possible. However, a way must be found to protect freedom of choice to have DNA analysis performed, without any negative social consequences. It must in any case be clear that the results of such analyses cannot be considered acceptable as a selection criterion for employment or insurance.

Conclusions

The availability of DNA analysis for families with a hereditary form of cancer represents a major extension of the diagnostic possibilities. The main importance of the analysis is that at-risk relatives of a patient can be spared the burdensome screening procedure. One of the disadvantages is that when the defective gene has been identified, the subject becomes aware of the chance that he or she may later develop cancer, and this may create a very difficult situation. Even though adequate treatment is available for most of the forms of cancer in question, the advantages and disadvantages must be weighed carefully before DNA analysis is performed. Freedom of choice is of prime importance for those involved in this decision. Detailed information and good psychosocial guidance are indispensable for the performance of such an analysis. Close collaboration between the clinical geneticists and the physicians responsible for follow-up of the families is an absolute requirement for the performance of DNA analysis. Because of the many problems associated with DNA analysis which can have various unanticipated consequences, much research is still to be done to define the psychosocial implications of preclinical and presymptomatic DNA diagnosis.

REFERENCES

1 McKusick VA: Mendelian inheritance in man. The Johns Hopkins University Press. Baltimore and London, 1990

2 Vasen HFA: Screening for hereditary tumours. Thesis, Utrecht 1989

3 Müller Hj and Vasen HFA: Prävention familiärer Tumorkrankheiten durch genetische Beratung und Frühdiagnostik. Schweiz Med Wschr 1990 (120):1451-1460

4 Tops CMJ, Griffioen G, Vasen HFA et al: Presymptomatic diagnosis of familial adenomatous polyposis by bridging DNA markers. The Lancet 1989 (2):1361-1363

5 Meera Khan P, van den Broek MH, Tops JMJ et al: Family studies in search of genes determining hereditary colorectal cancer. In: 5th International Symposium on Colorectal Cancer, Biology and Management of High Risk Groups. Elsevier Publishers, Amsterdam 1991 (in press)

6 Niermeyer MF: Eurogenetics 1989 - Das Program der Europäische Gemeinschaft. In: Sass H-M (ed) Genomanalyse und Gentherapie. Springer Verlag, Heidelberg 1991

7 Erfelijkheid: wetenschap en maatschappij. Over de mogelijkheden en grenzen van erfelijkheidsdiagnostiek en gentherapie. Adviescommissie van de Gezondheidsraad, 1989

UICC Strategy Meeting

Familial Cancer Among Cancer Patients Registered at the Aichi Cancer Registry - Heterogeneity of Aggregation of Familial Cancer

Kunio Aoki and Hiroshi Ogawa

Aichi Cancer Centre, Nagoya, Japan

Epidemiological studies on familial cancer may contribute to elucidate the causal mechanism of cancer - not only the genetic aspects, but also the role of environmental factors - because most cancers occurring in adulthood seem to depend on host and environmental interaction. The aim of this review is to disclose the role of the environment in familial cancer by looking at the heterogeneity of distribution, and to obtain information on familial aggregation for cancer control programmes. Most data in this paper derive from Ogawa's reports [1,2] on studies of familial cancer based on the Aichi Cancer Registry. A total of 9,131 registered cases in 1979-81 were analysed. In this paper, some data were reanalysed.

Heterogeneity of Familiy History in Cancer Patients by Site

A total of 9,131 cases (males 4,653, females 4,478) aged 20 years and older were examined. The proportion of cancer patients with a family history of cancer was 24.5% (male 24.4%, females 24.6%).

Table 1 shows the proportions of familial cancer cases by site and the calculated ratios of familial cancer rate to estimated average cancer mortality rate by site for the last 30 years. The proportion of patients with a family history was high for stomach cancer, 12.2%, while in other cancer types it ranged from 1.2 to 2.9%. The heterogeneous frequency of familial cancer in time and place seemed to be dependent on the impact of environmental factors on genetic conditions. Cancer incidence and mortality by site were different among areas and/or observed periods. The incidence of stomach cancer in Japan has been very high for the last 3 decades, despite of the recent declining trend, while cancer of the lung, colon and breast had a very low incidence in the 1950s, followed by a gradual increase up to the present [3]. The reason why average cancer mortality rates for the last decades were used in Table 1 is because the proportion of familial cancer at the moment seemed to be influenced by the cumulative numbers of patients from the past to the present. It may be noted that the ratios of familial cancer rate (A) to average mortality rate (B) did not show any significant difference among cancer sites, despite the high rate of familial cancer in stomach cancer. The slightly higher ratios for cancers of the colon-rectum may suggest that genetic factors play an important role in carcinogenesis. The slightly lower ratio for lung cancer may partly be due to the very low incidence in the 1950s.

Smoking and Familial History of Cancer

A case-control analysis was carried out to estimate the relative cancer risk in relation to family history and smoking habits [2]. The relative risk of lung cancer was 1.69 for those subjects with a family history alone, 2.23 for those with a smoking habit alone and 3.64 for those with both family history and smoking. This finding points to a synergistic action of factors. The contribution of family history to stomach cancer was moderate and the rela-

Table 1. Frequency (%) of familial cancer history in cancer patients registered at the Aichi Cancer Registry, Ogawa

	Percentages of pts with family history (A)	Average mortality* of cancer by site per 100,000 (B)	A to B
Stomach	12.2	65	0.2
Colon-Rectum	2.1	8	0.3
Liver	2.0	13	0.2
Lung	1.5	13	0.1
Breast	1.2	5	0.2
Uterus	2.9	15	0.2
All sites	24.5	14	0.2

* Roughly estimated

tive risk of family history for colon-rectum was more than 3.0. Smoking was shown to have almost no effect on the risk of stomach cancer, but was associated with a slightly elevated relative risk of uterine cancer and a modestly decreased risk of colorectal cancer. The risk of liver cancer was slightly influenced by both family history and smoking. When lung cancer was classified into 2 histological groups, adenocarcinoma was shown to be hardly affected by smoking, while the epidermoid type turned out to be closely related not only to smoking but also to family history (Fig. 1).

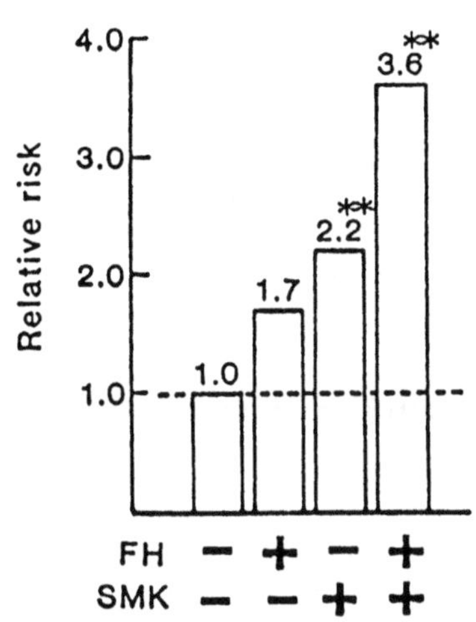

Fig. 1. Case-control analysis of lung cancer in relation to family history and smoking [a,b]

a) Mantel-Haenszel estimate adjusted for age and sex
b) Cases: lung cancer patients, controls: patients with cancer of sites other than the major sites
** $p<0.01$
FH Family history of lung cancer (+ = presence, - = absence)
SMK Smoking (+ = smoker and ex-smoker, - = never smoked)

Familial History and Lifestyle Habits Other than Smoking

The relative risk of stomach cancer was not affected by smoking, drinking and occupations such as the professions, management and skilled labour, but slightly elevated by occupations involving physical labour such as farming, fishing and others. The risk of colorectal cancer was increased by drinking and certain occupations (physical labour), but smoking was a suppressive factor. Marital status was shown not to be related to breast cancer risk. These results point to a certain heterogeneity in cancer risk according to site (Fig. 2).

Age Distribution of Cancer Patients With or Without Family History

Figure 3 shows the age distribution curves for colorectal and stomach cancer. Colorectal cancer with a family history of colorectal cancer showed a clear bimodal distribution which suggested the existence of 2 groups: a younger age group with high susceptibility and an older age group with ordinary susceptibility and stronger environmental influ-

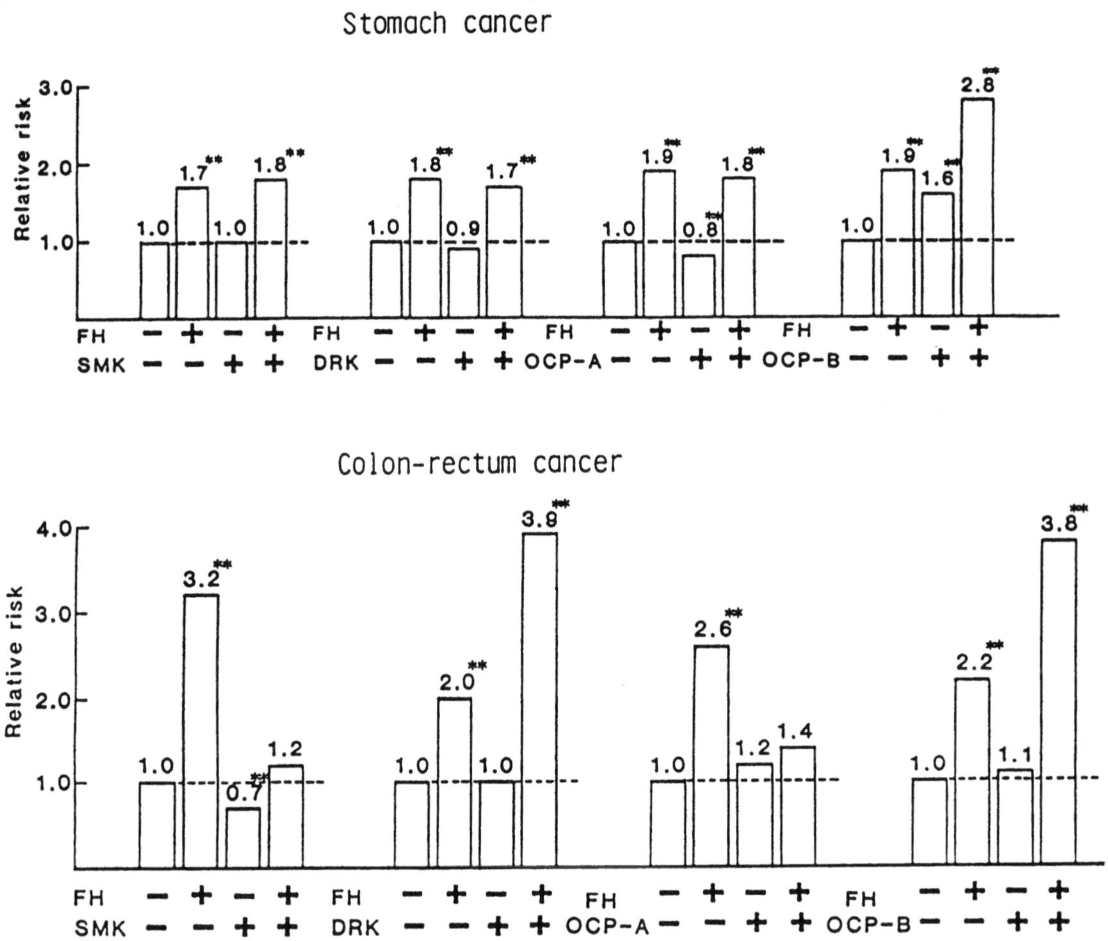

Fig. 2. Case-control analysis of cancers of the stomach and colon-rectum in relation to family history and lifestyle factors a,b

a) Mentel-Haenszel estimate adjusted for age and sex ($p<0.01$)
b) Controls: patients with cancer of sites other than stomach, colon, rectum, liver, lung, breast and uterus
FH Family history of stomach cancer for stomach cancer, or colorectal cancer for colorectal cancer patients (parents and siblings)
SMK Smoking (- = never smoker, + = smokers including ex-smokers)
DRK Alcohol consumer (- = non-drinker, + = regular drinker)
OCP Occupation A) professionals, managers, engineers etc.
B) farmers, fishermen, forest workers, labourers etc.

ence. The age distribution of cases without any family history of cancer showed a single peak at the age of 60-79.

On the other hand, no significant differences were observed in the age distribution of stomach cancer with or without family history, suggesting a lesser effect of familial factors on stomach cancer. These results strongly indicate that environmental factors play a substantial role in familial aggregation of cancer; the extent to which is dependent upon cancer site.

Discussion

Family members have undergone common exposure to environmental factors for long and it is natural that familial aggregation of cancer is closely related to environmental factors. However, the heterogeneity of the effects on cancer incidence should further be studied to establish effective ways of cancer prevention by controlling environmental factors.

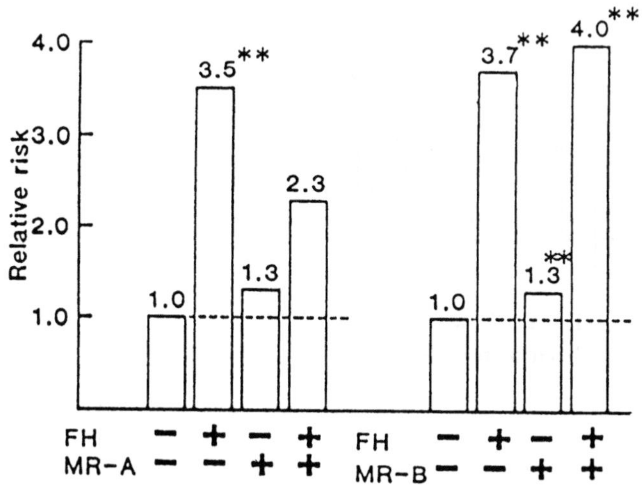

Fig. 3. Case-control analysis of breast cancer in relation to family history and marital status [a,b]

a) Mantel-Haenszel estimate adjusted for age and sex
b) Cases: breast cancer patients, controls: patients with cancer of sites other than the major sites
** $p<0.01$
FH Family history of breast cancer (+ = presence, - = absence)
MR-A Marital status (+ = single, - = others)
MR-B Marital status (+ = married, - = others)

REFERENCES

1 Ogawa H, Kato I and Tominaga S: Family history of cancer among cancer patients. Jpn J Cancer Res (Gann) 1985 (76): 113-118

2 Ogawa H, Tominaga S and Kato I: Family clustering of cancer: Analysis of cancer registry data. Gann Monogr on Cancer Res 1988 (35): 135-144

3 Kurihara M, Aoki and K, Hisamichi S (eds): Cancer Mortality Statistics in the World, 1950-1984. Univ of Nagoya Press, Nagoya, 1989

Report of the First UICC Strategy Meeting on Familial Cancer

W. Weber

Swiss Cancer League, Bern, Switzerland

Prof. M.M. Burger opens the meeting by presenting the UICC and its activities. He stresses that programmes have to generate their own money and asks the participants what they would like to do. The UICC is a vehicle for communication (e.g., ICPDES).

Prof. K. Aoki gives an overview of UICC epidemiology and prevention activities. He then presents the following guidelines for a prevention programme in familial cancer aggregations.

Step 1: Worldwide collection of scientific data (epidemiology, clinical pathology, molecular biology etc.) with the goal of creating a common terminology.

Step 2: Definition of risk factors directly connected with familial cancer aggregation.

Step 3: Finding effective means of cancer prevention.

A general discussion ensues in which the following points are put forward for consideration:

- Study psychosocial, ethical and legal aspects of familial cancer.
- Comparison between countries.
- Exchange of data and biological material of extended cancer families.
- Establishment and connection of familial cancer registries.
- Exchange of familial cancer researchers.
- Create units for family studies.
- Examine family study strategies.
- Initiate the family study approach.
- Offer expertise to beginners.
- Promote international collaboration.
- Involve nurses.
- Concentrate on one frequent tumour. Focus on the most prominent feature.
- Computerise family data.
- Introduce family data into ongoing studies.
- Encourage existing groups and foundations to organise transdisciplinary courses and meetings.
- Study malformations and cancer.
- Study environmental courses of familial cancer clustering.

The following aims were set at this first meeting:

1. Establish a uniform code sheet and guidelines for collecting family data.
2. Establish definitions, standards, a common terminology and methodology.
3. Collect data at different levels of definition.
4. Write a manual on the Family Study Unit.
5. Make a directory of Familial Cancer Study Groups.
6. Organise Familial Cancer Strategy Meetings for Asia, Oceania and America in 1992.
7. Organise a UICC International Familial Cancer Meeting in Switzerland in 1993.

The Swiss Cancer League is offering support for preparatory activities until 1993; it is hoped that a UICC programme or project can be established within this time course.

Subject Index